MIND, AYURVEDA & YOGA PSYCHOLOGY

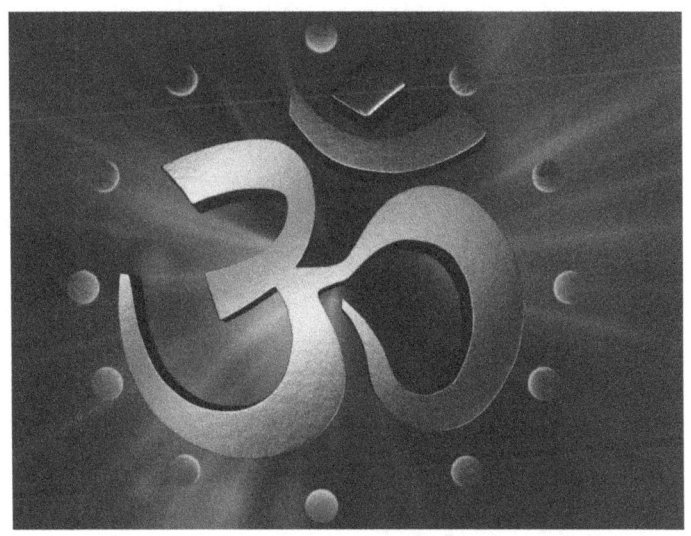

Dr. John Cosby

FAMILY PHYSICIAN
& AYURVEDA PRACTITIONER

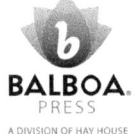

BALBOA
PRESS
A DIVISION OF HAY HOUSE

Copyright © 2017 Dr. John Cosby.

All rights reserved. No part of this book may be used or reproduced by any means, graphic, electronic, or mechanical, including photocopying, recording, taping or by any information storage retrieval system without the written permission of the author except in the case of brief quotations embodied in critical articles and reviews.

This book is a work of non-fiction. Unless otherwise noted, the author and the publisher make no explicit guarantees as to the accuracy of the information contained in this book and in some cases, names of people and places have been altered to protect their privacy.

Balboa Press books may be ordered through booksellers or by contacting:

Balboa Press
A Division of Hay House
1663 Liberty Drive
Bloomington, IN 47403
www.balboapress.com
1 (877) 407-4847

Because of the dynamic nature of the Internet, any web addresses or links contained in this book may have changed since publication and may no longer be valid. The views expressed in this work are solely those of the author and do not necessarily reflect the views of the publisher, and the publisher hereby disclaims any responsibility for them.

The author of this book does not dispense medical advice or prescribe the use of any technique as a form of treatment for physical, emotional, or medical problems without the advice of a physician, either directly or indirectly. The intent of the author is only to offer information of a general nature to help you in your quest for emotional and spiritual well-being. In the event you use any of the information in this book for yourself, which is your constitutional right, the author and the publisher assume no responsibility for your actions.

Any people depicted in stock imagery provided by Thinkstock are models, and such images are being used for illustrative purposes only. Certain stock imagery © Thinkstock.

Print information available on the last page.

ISBN: 978-1-5043-8311-0 (sc)
ISBN: 978-1-5043-8326-4 (e)

Balboa Press rev. date: 08/02/2017

Contents

Preface.. vii
Acknowledgments.. xiii
Introduction..xv

Part 1: The Function of Mind
Chapter 1: Mind (Manas) 1
Chapter 2: Samkhya Philosophy 17
Chapter 3: The Three Gunas: Sattva, Rajas,
　　　　　　and Tamas 32

Part 2: Yoga Psychology
Chapter 4: Yoga Psychology.......................................41
Chapter 5: Ashtanga Yoga:
　　　　　　The Eightfold Path of Yoga 55
Chapter 6: Asana and Pranayama:
　　　　　　The Science of Postures and Breath.......74
Chapter 7: Thoughtless Meditation 94

Part 3: The Science of Ayurveda
Chapter 8: Tridosha: Prakriti and Vikriti 117
Chapter 9: Ayurveda: Digestion
　　　　　　and Sapta Dhatus 147
Chapter 10: Ayurveda and Mental Health............... 164
Chapter 11: Diet for Vatta, Pitta, and Kapha........... 174
Chapter 12: Gunas and Foods 196
Chapter 13: Ayurvedic Herbs for the Mind............. 201
Chapter 14: Asanas for Vata, Pitta, and
　　　　　　 Kapha Constitutions............................223

Part 4: Integrating the Yoga Traditions
Chapter 15: Karma, Bhakti,
      Raja, and Jnana Yogas..........................235
Chapter 16: Conclusion 247

Bibliography..261
Autobibliography...263

Preface

The year was 1975, and the girl next to me in the church choir kept telling me her sister taught meditation and that I should meet her. I had never sung in the choir before, but I found myself placed in the second tenor section surrounded by some talented individuals. I had settled on the Pentacostal church because of the sincerity and passion of the pastor's speeches toward his aspiring congregation. After I was told this several times over four Sundays, I spontaneously said I would meet her sister that day. After church we took the New York City subway three train stops before exiting to the street to walk four blocks to her sister's apartment. I figured the visit would be a courteous one with a brief introduction and more chatter, and then I'd be on my way. Inside her older sister's apartment, I waited with ease on the couch for her to emerge from the rear bedroom. After several minutes, she came down the hallway and appeared at the living room entrance. I remember the effulgent aura she exuded from her whole persona while she stood near where I was sitting. Her hair glowed with softness. Her skin was bright and lustrous, and her eyes danced and sparkled with a shining light. She appeared absolutely calm and content with her surroundings. At the time I did not know what an aura was, but I sensed something was being generated from her physical boundary. Whatever it was, I knew I wanted her state of serenity. That was Sunday afternoon.

By the following Friday (five days later), I returned to her sister's apartment. This time I was going to be initiated into meditation. I would be given a mantra sound to meditate on. Although I did not know what meditation was, I did remember reading that while touring India, the four legendary Beatles from England had been initiated into transcendental meditation by the Maharishi Mahesh Yogi. That was the extent of my knowledge other than it supposedly made you calm and you exuded peace. Before arriving I was instructed to bring several fragrant flowers, one coconut, three fruits, and incense sticks for the preparation of a *puja*. Puja is the ritual ceremony where you receive instructions on the sound of mantra before beginning the practice of meditation. The puja initiation is an ancient and sacred Hindu ritual, attuned by the provocation of root sounds to energize the sound of the mantra into your unconscious and conscious mind. The power of the mantra creates a snowball effect of the inestimable number of initiates who have recited the sound over many centuries. The root of the mantra is derived from the Sanskrit language, which is recognized as the oldest and purest phonetic sound used today.

The scenario of a puja was foreign to me, as I had no idea what meditation was or what one should feel. All I knew at that point was my sixteen years of ingrained Catholic school beliefs (grade school, high school and university levels) that prepared me for another vocation within the walls of the church. Regardless of my earlier concepts, I instinctively knew deep down this was the beginning of a major transformation in my life, one that would lead me on my journey in search of an answer to the universal question about who I really was. I sensed something mystical that was beyond my imagination and relative intellect was about to take place. So I intuitively went ahead with performing the puja, and I opened up with no anticipation to explore the awaiting unknown experience.

In puja, I was given a mantra root word—a mystical incantation—by her sister. She softly whispered the strange sound into my ear. The mantra sound was not like anything I had heard before. It was a gentle vibration and comforting sound that immediately felt right inside me. It innately vibrated inside, and I instinctively trusted that. She repeated it several times until I got the hang of the new Sanskrit mantra sound, which I could effortlessly and silently repeat within me.

The puja consisted of three consecutive days of practicing the mantra sound. Each day was basically the same practice setup as to the other two, but what I experienced each time was something beyond words. Repeating this vibrating mantra softly again and again with eyes closed, in a short span of time, spontaneously expanded my inner awareness. Intuitively, I drifted further and further away from my collection of thoughts and instead experienced more silence and oneness with the expansion of consciousness. It was like an atomic bomb blast that shoots upward and outward in a mushroom cloud and spreads endlessly away from the site of the explosion and beyond. Instead it was my consciousness that kept expanding infinitely with the sound of the mantra. I had become one with it without any effort. There were no thoughts and concepts attached to the outward exploration, just the ongoing expansion of consciousness. The experience was unlike anything I could have possibly imagined before that day. It was powerful, gentle, soothing, and not upsetting in any way. The experience of the whispered mantra would leave a profound mark on my consciousness and the way I would view my relationships, surrounding circumstances, and myself. It gave me the subtle realization about exactly what I needed to work toward because I now had direction of purpose to where I wanted to go.

By looking back over the number of years that life has given me, it is the moment when I was introduced to mantra meditation that I give the most credence and substance to in my life. That first puja initiation experience gave rise to a major life-changing experience. It was a mystical experience that went beyond words and intellect. The experience kindled a spontaneous expansion of my core personality into infinite waves that kept moving and moving with no finite or confined boundaries. The experience was breathtaking, and it ignited a spark of consciousness within that has continued to grow greater over the years. The seed was planted in the soil, and it would sprout and grow into a huge mango tree.

Up to that point in my life, I was never taught how to experience different levels consciousness. This was definitely not something I would learn in high school, university, church, and at home with my parents. After the experience I knew deep down inside me that this would somehow stretch me and help me search inside to who I really was. Things would have to change in my life if I continued to meditate on the mantra sound.

After the experience of being initiated into the sound mantra meditation, I started to explore books on anything that related to meditation. I found myself reading as many books on the topics of thoughts, mind, meditation, and consciousness. I was drawn toward books on Eastern philosophy and yoga, many urged the need to change how one thought to work towards the control of mind in order to reach higher levels of consciousness. I needed more than books to expand the experience of daily meditation. Thus, found myself frequently attending group meditation sessions, which were more energetic and deeper in experience. This led me to the regular practice of yoga, meditation, and breathing exercises, all of which solidified the lifestyle that I was embracing. Thus, it is the gainful experiences over the years and the significant changes in spiritual personality that have inspired me to write this book for others about the power of thought and mind.

Acknowledgments

I wish to give special thanks to Sri Swami Jyotirmayananda (Yoga Research Foundation, Miami, Fl) for his wisdom and intuitive intellect into the mysticism of the sacred scriptures; his display of tireless and selfless service to others; and the compassion, devotion, and love he pours on those who meet him in the satsanga hall. His insightfulness of the scriptures has inspired many over the decades to achieve greater spiritual growth through the knowledge of the Vedas. The inner glow of his light continues to shine brighter on those that come his way to gain knowledge of the ancient scriptures. *Om Tat Sat.*

Also, Dr. Vasant Lad, renown Ayurveda physician, who encouraged and inspired me into the science of Ayurveda for the healing of self and others.

I would like to give special warmth, love, and affection to my children, Desiree and Yohannan, and also to my best friend, Dhumakesha (spiritual buddy of thirty years), whose dancing eyes sparkle with her bright smile and laughter, affect everyone around her. Her genuine personality exudes boundless joy, love, and compassion to others around her.

Kannika Leanarch... ...my panraya......the love of my life.

Introduction

The pull on the individual psyche to the external is greater today than at any time in the history of the human race. The bombardment of ever-changing, hi-tech instruments overloading our psyche is progressing with greater speed and a vastness of stimuli, and all this prompts hasty decision making the mind's intellect and reason to act faster. The overwhelming impact of the subliminal messages of marketing strategies has designed the capacity to go beyond our natural ability to adapt and safeguard the mind from being overworked. The split signals the loss of our inner identities to the world of objectivity. This constant bombardment has had detrimental effects on the very core of our personalities. These ill effects, manifested as psychosomatic disorders, have shown up in significant numbers at clinics and hospitals through the past two decades. It seems everyone knows someone with signs and symptoms of distress, anxiety, panic attacks, nervousness, cardiac arrhythmia, chest tightness, shortness of breath, insomnia, or depression.

Much of modern medicine, including primary-care physicians and psychiatrists, has been overwhelmed by the demands to instantly heal the increasing society mental ills, even to the point of prescribing heavy and toxic medicines, such as antipsychotic, anxiolytic, and anti-depressive drugs. All of these are intended to neutralize the onslaught on the mind. These psychiatric drugs are prescribed at high dosages—one, two, and four hundred milligrams—and we are supposed to take them throughout the day and at bedtime. How does one function on such heavy regimens?

But what is lacking is a higher and subtler dimension of reality that treads beyond our physical world. We need to research consciousness beyond our limited laboratories. Consciousness cannot be touched or examined physically in laboratories. The brain can be tested with electrode devices to identify areas that connect to speech and vision. Yes, the hippocampus is the region of the brain that facilitates emotion and memory. But it has difficulty to explain how memory store impressions and later merge ino thought to be acted on. The mind and brain are two different entities. It's the mind that facilitates the operation of the brain and the entire nervous system in the body. The physical brain through its circuitry allows the input of sensory impressions from the outer. But it is the mind that digests the outside stimuli, which enables us humans to interrelate with others and the objective world. It's the mind that needs to be explored through the paradigm of consciousness to realize how the different functions of the mind operate as one not individually. Is there a universal source that allows the mind to shine and see the external and internal impressions that appears in our lives?

Most agree that the mind controls the body. The mind uses the instrument of the senses and body consciousness to come alive so we perceive those and objects around us. It is the operative mind that project the functions of intellect, memory, and ego to give one the capacity to interrelate and experience the relative world. The practical world of getting a higher degree of education, raising a family and working for a living are important aspects of life. On a higher spiritual level, the mind is able to transform into rays of illuminated consciousness which mirrors the greater sum of pure consciousness that permeates everything to play its part in the universes.

In this book we will help to explain the mind and its relationship within the field of consciousness. We will view the concepts of consciousness and mind in the form of the ancient texts of India. These ancient texts, known as the Vedas, are several thousand years old and have proven the test of time. The source of this profound knowledge in consciousness was derived from the seers and sages who intuitively experienced and realized that everything was explicable to the expansion of consciousness. These layers of infinite consciousness were refractions of the non-attributes of pure consciousness (creative force) that lies beneath the manifestation of everything in the cosmos, whether it be the macrocosm (universe) or the microcosm (man).

With its vast literature on human and cosmic consciousness, the Vedic tradition offers a compelling store of information on the nature of the mind and how our thoughts determine our patterns of daily life. The existence of every thought and its related action creates one's present and future circumstances, whether positive and negative, pleasurable and painful. We have the power to change and shape our thoughts through the many yogic sciences to improve the mental processes of ourselves. Through concentration methods we can narrow our thoughts to one-pointedness to become more still and attentive in our minds. The practice of mantra meditation to allow us to tap into the depth of the mind where an absolute silence or residual potential space lies. There have been popular books written that talk about reaching our full potential and changing the way we think to subconsciously design our world. And they are not wrong. It is true—the full potential of the mind is hidden and needs to be explored, but merely knowing this is not necessarily effective in changing the way we think and respond in our daily activities that are being altered constantly. For most of us, we need to have someone who has mastered the mind or can be shown steps to gradually centered the mind to become attentive and directive in whatever we set out to do.

The Veda holds the most data on the aspects of the mind, and it offers a myriad of practical disciplines—asanas (postures), pranayama (control of breath), one-pointed-concentration, deep meditation, and control the mind. The control of thought and mind has the power to make or break your world because thoughts alone create how you see yourself and relationship to circumstances. You are the captain of your ship and your destiny. Only 10 percent of our awakening consciousness is used by the conscious mind. The remaining 90 percent is left to the operative subconscious and unconscious. Without insight into the hidden workings of the subconscious and unconscious mind, one is left defenseless to the waves of relentless circumstances affronting us daily. This is the advantage of doing the regular practice of any yogic principles discussed later in the book, which offers you to begin to integrate through awareness the interplay of the conscious and unconscious mind so that they become balanced and create harmony in your mental state.

So what is unique about this book? I will seek to share with you the most important psychological principles of the ancient traditions. The most important aspect of all human life lies in the mind. The mind alone is the conscious faculty of the brain capable of perceiving itself and the surrounding world. No other creature on our planet has the ability to do so. The human mind has engineered the tallest buildings, built huge cruise ships to cross the oceans, built powerful weapons, and made spaceships to travel to distant planets. It can experience emotions of happiness and sadness, love and hatred, and anger and calm. It has the capacity to intellectualize and reason complex mathematics and science dilemmas. On a psychological level, the mind has the ability to change its concepts and beliefs in order to better or worse its circumstances. It can adapt to the stresses of life by shifting its attention to overcome adversity to bring calm to the mind. On a spiritual level, one can explore the inner world and discover their full residual potential and realize the innate nature of themselves.

Many never reach their full potential. They fall

short and only change superficially to themselves and external things. They get caught up into the pull of the theatrical stage of life. Life appears to be a whirlpool, and each day brings new issues that have to be tackled, leaving little growth of the inner self. Sadly, we do not know where to begin or how to go about it. No one has ever taught us how to slow the mind down or how to empower thoughts, to better the direction our thoughts can respond to life situations. One's desires, cravings, sentiments, and instincts are buried deep in the unconscious mind. The unconscious can strongly influence and direct one's perception, memory, ego, intellect, and reason to the point we act (unknowing) in a certain way. If left to itself, there is no real transformation of personality and spiritual growth. The unconscious mind is not accessible for many, simply because the conscious mind has no awareness of it. Its not for trying but just not knowing. We need to become more aware to the influence and workings of the unconscious mind.

The unconscious mind begins to build up data when the conscious mind passes through the stages in childhood and adulthood to gather impressions of enjoyments, achievements, frustration, conflict, and all sorts of experiences that leave their psychological markings on the recorded device beneath the mind.

These impressions are formed at the time the mind perceives them, and simultaneously stored in the unconscious. The unconscious perceives the incoming impression without any bias to right and wrong. There the impressions lie in the depth of the unconscious until they arise to the waking field of the conscious mind to perform their dance on the world stage. The unconscious mind is nothing but a collection of seeded impressions—habits, instincts, desires, feelings, ideas, and concepts. In the fertile unconscious field, they begin to sprout and grow to maturity. At maturity these impressions (i.g, unresolved feelings) coexist in the conscious mind and together play out in thought, speech, and action.

Here is where the psychology of yoga (self-analysis) offers one the necessary knowledge to become aware of the power of thought and its subsequent action. Through yogic disciplines, we learn how to rise above the mountains of thoughts that burden our vision and see what is on the other side. We can become aware of the rise and fall of thought waves, and how these impressions are formed by partial feeling, thought, and reason. We can learn to navigate the force of thoughts that either support better choices or hold us back. We can learn to develop the ability to quiet thoughts in order to improve our mental personality. To achieve these seemingly arduous tasks, yogic philosophies have broken down the spiritual journey into numerous practical steps to bring us to explore and find what is compatible to them.

The book is divided into four parts: 1) Function of Mind 2) Yoga Psychology 3) Science of Ayurveda, and 4) Integrating the Yoga Tradition.

In the *first part of this book*, we will look at some of

the foundational concepts of several yogic philosophies, especially one's pertaining to the nature of the mind. We will look at the structure, and characteristics of the mind. The different functions of the mind - senses, feelings, ego, memory, and intellect - and the interchange of them to form thought and consequently influence what direction the mind moves and acts. We will show how the mind has the capacity to ascend to the higher mind (clarity, tranquility, intuitive intelligence), or descend to the realm of the lower mind (faulty, habitual, instinctive thinking). In chapter two, Samkhya philosophy is illustrated to explain the enfolding creation in the expression of everything throughout our universe. For the purpose of this book, we will pay more attention to the evolutionary process of the cosmic mind to the progression of individual intelligence. It is at this stage that the conjunction of individual intelligence and ego originates into the process of the human mind. Of importance, we will discuss the significance of the ego factors in relation to sattva (pure, harmony), rajas (activity, passion), and tamas (substance, inertia) and the mind. We will discuss the interplay between the three gunas in terms of the tendencies and qualities of each and their impact on the mind, and how they influence the shape and color of perception of the individual self and the surrounding world.

In the third chapter of part one, we will further the discussion of the three gunas (universal qualities, tendencies). The existence of the three gunas are present in all beings and objects, and in turn, give working expression to them. On a psychological level, they give rise to the many personalities traits of man which will be further detailed in the book.

In the *second part of the book,* yoga psychology, we will look at practical disciplines within the various yoga schools to rise above the mental tides of agitation and despair to higher ground of intuitive intelligence and reason. In particular, we will look at the Yoga Sutras of Patanjali, which end point is to cease all distracted movement of thoughts, in order to achieve total control of the mind. Patanjali outlines eight disciplines which can be implemented into our lives to quiet and silent the mind to reach the ultimate goal in self-realization. We will also examine the mental afflictions in the form of the five *kleshas* – ignorance, ego, attachment, aversion and hatred, and clinging to fear, doubt and death - which cause impediments to the advancement of one's spiritual growth. The overlapping of the five kleshas are the basis of all human pain, misery and suffering. You can think of the five kleshas as robbers that take your virtiuos qualities from the domain of your mind.

In the *third part of the book*, we will look at the science of ayurveda as a comprehensive, holistic health care system that supports the intrinsic nature of both mental and bodily health. This is a practical healing science and together with the yogic philosophies, helps to integrate the spiritual personality. The ultimate goal of ayurveda is to maintain good health of body and mind and restore the homeostasis of the body in times of illness and disease. We will also discuss the ayurveda theory of the three doshas - vata, pitta, and kapha—three energetic forces that circulate and govern the entire physiological activities in the body. Ayurveda emphasize the equilibrium between the three doshas, in order to sustain balance and health of the physiopsychological state of the individual. These bio-elements (or doshas) are constantly changing in response to internal feelings, thoughts, emotions, distresses, and external forces of foods, weather, and seasons. In essence, when people live within their intrinsic nature of existence, is there balance between the doshas and vice versa. We will take an indepth look at the science of nutrition (ayurveda) that offers an effective approach to the balance of the dosha(s) to achieve health. Ayurveda's huge database on food substance over the centuaries, has categorizes what is appropriate to eat or not eat to nourish the three dosha body types of the individual. In conjunction, it recognizes the importance of a strong gastric fire to properly digest food, and breakdown large ingested substance to viable micro-nourishment to feed the miniscule seven tissues (structure and function), and to cleanse by expel of waste and toxins from the body.

In *part four of the book*, integrating the yoga traditions, we will show the integration of karma, bhakti, raja, and jnana yoga correlation to the balance of the four aspect of the human personality – action, emotion, will, and wisdom. The integration of one's personality depends upon a balanced and harmonious development of these aspects. The Yoga-process is one's integral process, but named differently accordingly to its specialized emphasis. The Yoga that trains reason is known as Jnana Yoga or Yoga of Wisdom. The Yoga that develops blazing love of God and causes emotional integration is called Bhakti Yoga or Yoga of Devotion. The Yoga that enables one to control the mind through meditation is called Raja Yoga. The Yoga that enables one to prepare his psychological being to face and confront the day-to-day activities of life, and also unfolds his hidden potentialities is called Karma Yoga, the Yoga of Action.

Together, ayurvedic and yogic traditions offer profound and powerful insights into the nature, cause, and cure of mental and bodily afflictions. They also offer an array of practices for achieving the optimum state of individual health. In this book you will find an integral approach to numerous practices and philosophies of yogic systems and the science of Ayurveda, and it's my hope that these will be of tremendous assistance on your personal path to enlightenment.

Part 1: The Function of Mind

Chapter 1: Mind (Manas)

Introduction

In this chapter, I will provide you with information as it specifically pertains to the working of the mind. We will cover the subject of the nature, structure, and characteristics of the mind. We will look at the four functions of mind, intellect, ego, memory and how collectively they organize thought that lead to action and experience. The interplay of the four functions are not separate but act together as one to undertake the mental activities of the mind. We will discuss the concept of the higher self (purity, clarity and tranquility) and lower self (agitation and confusion). The mind alone has the ability to pursue either the spiritual higher mind, or be drawn down to the lower state of mind - associated with the senses and body consciousness.

The Nature of Mind (Sanskrit-Word Manas)

The mind is extremely active, mobile, subtle, and difficult to control. The mind is ever-changing. The mind is restless and energetic of pepertual thoughts. It very seldom stays in one place. It likes to move from one situation to another for interest and enjoyment. If allowed, it will move in every direction without resistance and restraints. The mind seems so vast and diverse because of the perpetual change in direction to the unlimited number of perceived objects it can sense, digest, differentiate, and categorization of them. Its nature is to form differences, separation and division of the external world. It is a series of changing points of awareness without stop. The mind cannot attend to more than one thing at a time. There is constant change and direction to where the mind wants to go. When the mind stays focus does it gather information for the presence and absence of knowledge.

No other organ of the body can restrain the mind. Only mind can control itself. Mind controls the lower senses and body. Each of the five senses can only perform one function at a time. They are separate from one another. They do not coordinate with each other. The eyes only see, ears only hear, tongue only taste, nose only smell, and skin only feel. They function alone. Whereas, the mind is able to blend and direct the movement of all of the five senses.

The mind precedes the body. The mind commands the body to move in the direction it wants to go. When you are taking steps forward to begin running, your right and left leg are not deciding the action, but rather it is the action of thought that commands these intentional and well coordinated leg movements.

The objective form is the outer manifestation of the subjective mind. The material world accessed through the instruments of the senses is then perceived by the mind to give sensation to the object. The mind then attaches feeling (sense of being real) to the outer manifestation of the object. The perception of the outer is further processed by memory to compare past recognition or association of the objective form. The image-maker of ego enters to pigment (personal touch) the outer manifestation to how it sees and wants to act to the object. The faculty of intelligence then provides reason and comprehension to the objective image which then precipitates into thought form to arise so that one is able to experience the outer manifestation of their world.

The Structure of Mind

The mind is neither outside nor inside. It is without shape and size. It appears to be without structure, and it lacks the physical structure of the body. Mind is the subtle form of matter in our physical world. The mind is swifter and lighter than the heavier and structured contents of the body. While the physical body is fixated in time and space, the subtle mind lies beyond the dimensions of our physical world. Its existence lies within the astral plane. The mental processes operate at unimaginable speed to be recorded. Over the centuries the scholars have tried to understand how the mind works. But the mind remains a mystery organ even to the current scientific laboratory findings. It cannot be touched and dissected in the laboratory. Modern science has tried to map lobe regions of the brain with electrodes to explore the many activities of the mind. They have found observable energies and related intangible expressions of them, but fail to exlain the source of the structure and location of the mind. The best laboratory is the mind. The need to reflect, enquire, and witness is essential to the exploration of the inner identity of the mind. One must go beyond the sphere of the mind to realize there is no structure and location but rather consciousness alone which the ancient philosophies and wisdom of the sages knew all along.

Matter of Mind

The mind is the cause of everything that manifests in your world. The world you create to live in is nothing but a collection of impressions – instincts, habits, feelings, perceptions, desires, ambitions, ideas – generated by the walking mind. These thoughts when not in use in the present state of wakefulness are lost to the unconscious mind. They lay hidden in the unconscious while waiting to arise to the surface of the waking state in response to some problems, expectations, anticipations, innovations, changing conditions, and growth in life.

The person in the waking state develop concepts to give identity of self and the exterior. The individual may see themselves as belonging to a particular family, born on a particular date, association to type of friends, personal relationships and family, social activities, pride of nation, and types of school that all together helped them learn how to challenge the daily experiences that life presents to you. They see themselves being drawn to different external factors of happiness and contentment, and development of antipathy toward feelings of unhappy and discomfort.

Mind, Ayurveda & Yoga Psychology

The waking world is unable to be touched and grasped, in that it stretches beyond the individual's physical presence, without consideration of the person. At times, the person appears to free fall like the leaf descending from the tree. The person may even feel they have no control to the world around them. The person feels duty-bound to the inestimable conditions imposed upon them by the objective world. The need to change is never taught to us on how to quiet, discipline and regulate the alternate wave movement of thought that seem to continually fill the mind.

In the waking state (Jagrat), the sense organs (indriyas) perceive the object of sense and relay the perception of the objective to the mind. The gross perceptions of the senses are simultaneously engaged by the mind (manas) which is sent to the faculty of the intellect (buddhi) to evaluate and filter the gross into subtler perceptions of information. But before the decision of the subtle perception is finalized does the ego factor enter the mental process to influence and pigment its agender of "mine-ness" into shaping the concluding information. The processed of subtle perception becomes an important source of knowledge in the waking state (although it is not the only source of knowledge).

In the waking state, the dominance influence of the ego factor subjugates the other mental functions - perception, feelings, intellect, reason and comprehension - to how the organization of thought is to be developed and projected in action. It wants to be the controller over others and situations in making decision and the acts of them. The impure nature of ego wants to breed selfishness, separation, ownership, anger, greed, jealousy, and arrogance that effects the process of thinking and speech. In summary, ego attires the mental functions that cause pain, sorrow, grief, and frustration to lead to experiences of disharmony in one's daily activities.

The ego is a wave movement that thread the fabric of attributes to thought. The ego-factor underlies thought and desires, thus it projects and sustains the realities of the waking state.

Its with the cultivation of thoughts that yoga psychology has given the most importance to the experiences of the waking state. The science of yoga realized the perception generated by the waking mind had a direct impact of those impressions seeded into the fertile ground of the unconscious mind, whether good and bad. The images and experience stored in the unconscious in turn made their way to the surface of the waking state when needed to give expression to act in the outer world. The philosophy of yoga recognized that change was needed to the formation of thought so to modify the past experiences of events and the thinking that now appear in one's daily activities.

According to many of the schools of yogic thought, the mind is made up of four major functions that play an essential role to the formation of thought. The four aspects of the mind as a whole is often referred as the internal instrument (antahkarana) of the mind. The four internal instruments are not separate but act together as one to undertake the mental activities of the mind to rise into thought form and knowledge. It is the integration of the four functions that allows perception, feeling, memory, ego, intelligence to arise thought into knowledge to understand the activities in his and her life.

Formation of Thought

In the Yoga Sutra of Patanjali, the four internal instruments of the mind are categorized as conscious mind (manas), intellect (buddhi), ego (ahamkara) and memory (smrti). Although they appear to be separate from one another, it is the coordinated confluence of the four instruments that unifies perception into thought, knowledge and experience of the world we live in.

The conscious (wake) mind is the objective mind. It thinks of objects. The intellect of mind gives reason and discrimination to objects. The ego is the self arrogate principle of mind. Smrti (chitta) is the storehouse of past impressions of the unconscious mind. Although it appears the process of thinking in the waking state plays a major role in perception of the present realities, it is the vast storage of past impressions and images of the unconscious that significantly imposes itself on how the conscious mind will think and operate in action. For most, around 10 percent of the waking state is used in the process of thinking to organize thought into information. The remaining 90 percent is left to the hidden operative unconscious mind. If there is little or no insight into the unseen workings of the unconscious mind, one is left defenseless to the waves of relentless circumstances affronting our waking existence.

Manas is the human mind, and its task is to think and facilitate knowledge. It is the inner organ of perception. It is interconnected to the outer through the projections of the five senses. The movement of impressionable content(s) taken into the mind is then processed to form cognition, comprehension, reason and intention in order for the individual mind to interrelate to the outer world.

Mind is the existence of the countless thoughts that is entertain in a life span. Thoughts become alive when mind assumes the form of an object and intensifies the content of that thought. If it thinks of an orange it takes on the form – color, shape, taste, sensation, and feel - of it. The thought that you hold onto becomes manifested in your life. Thoughts of compassion, kindness, joy, happiness and anger, greed and vanity will manifest in your physical world. The interplay of thought transgresses throughout one's life span unless change is undertaken.

Buddhi literally translates to awakened intelligence. It is through the intelligence faculty of buddhi that things are known, understood and identified. It gathers information to differentiate false from real. Its function is to accurately discriminate, evaluate, analyze, organize, and make decision.

Mind, Ayurveda & Yoga Psychology

Buddhi is the higher aspect of the mind. The higher mind (buddhi) of individual intelligence resonates the qualities of truth, positivity, clearness, and ingenuity. In its natural state, it operates daily activities in clear thinking, innate wisdom, judiciousness in decision making, and astute reason in the formation of knowledge. The mind is left to spontaneously move towards the direction of intuitive intelligence, brightness in discernment and judgement, and assimilate clear feeling and understanding. In this state of clearness, the mind is able to vision with accuracy the externalization as it really appears to be. The movement of the higher mind is drawn towards righteousness and selflessness in thought and action to others. It exudes brightness and positivity to the surrounding atmosphere. Others are effected by its exuberant personality.

Then there's the limited intellect that is dominated by faulty knowledge. The unclear information misleads the individual intelligence to act unsoundly in reason and comprehension. The mind is veiled by the cloudy shade of partiality which results in diminished clarity and vision. The mind becomes more tangled with its ideas, and widens in imagination. The mind is left with distractions in trying to make coherent decision to bring some matter to a conclusion (personal relationships). The mind grows in doubt and falls to poor decisions in life situations. The confused state of mind stretches itself to search for solutions to reinforce a sense of purpose in one's life. It's like the bee that goes endlessly from flower to flower in search of nectar. Similarly, the mind goes from object to object in search of solutions but comes up empty-handed, which leaves it search of new information to no end.

Ahamkara or ego is the part of the mind that intercedes the conscious and unconscious. The wave of ego-thought gives the sense of personal identity to the image of the individual. The faculty of egoism portrays your individual "I" identity. Its the self-asserting principle of the thinking faculty of mind. The imperceptible ego influences the mind to spread its feelings of affection (likes) and aversion (dislike), and happiness and sadness (duality). Thus, the faculty of ego creates differences and separation between the externalization and mind. The mind begins to take on the behavior of the ego in seeing everything as separate of itself. The ego wants to exert its power over object, relationship, and circumstances. The indiscernible ego wants recognition for its cleverness, and prides itself on doing a job well done. The ego will proclaim its stockpile of desires, needs, feelings, and ideas to those near and far away. It does not take to offense well and retort to ways to get back at the mistaken remarks of others. It blames others for its failure and mishaps.

The mind falls to the lower realm of thinking when it entertains to thoughts like "I am well educated, I am more important, I have many things, I know better, and You are wrong". The false identification of ego influences the way one thinks. The fabrication of ego tightens its grip on the activities of the ever changing mind. The mind is pulled away from the strength of its inner core and led to the enjoyment of the material world. The will of the influential ego accustoms the mind to thinking the daily adversities that happen outside of itself as normal. The illusiveness of ego moves the mind to fall victim to fear, doubt, vanity, importance, negative feeling and imagination, which vaccinates into the never-ending dramatic scenarios in one's life (not unlike soap operas).

The brightness of one's intelligence is overcome by the cloudy radiance of the false ego. The innate ability of the intellect to make sound reason and decision is compromise by the stronger expression of ego. The higher intelligence now plays second fiddle to the self-interest of the challenger and dominance of ego. The false ego colors and shapes the intellect to what flavors and tastes it wants to enjoy. The cunningness of ego changes one's perceptions from seeing what is real.

There are two aspects to the ego factor or the "I-identity". There's the virtuous ego factor, which moves one's mind in the direction of the highest self. The higher mind is bequeathed with right perception and clarity of intelligence. The healthy personality of the higher mind characterizes goodness, honesty, friendliness, and compassion. It sees itself as a part of the whole creation. The other ego factor is affiliated to the negative contents of the individual personality. It raises the notion of mine and ownership. It spawns the sense of possessiveness. The nature of selfishness begets the mind to focus on satisfying its self-interest.

Dr. John Cosby

It sees itself as separate from others. Others are means to advance their justifiable agenda or duty of interest. This separatism helps create the thought of duality in subjectivity and objectivity. If allowed to go on, the self-centered ego subjects the mind to intensify thinking in afflictions of pride, arrogance, competitiveness, greediness, and vanity.

Smriti refers to the storage of memory. It is the memory faculty of mind. It is one of the four functions of the internal instruments, antahkarana. The primary function of smriti is to store the past impressions in feelings, thoughts, attitudes, situations, and experiences collected by the preceptor of the waking mind. Although these past impressions appear to have faded when the waking mind turns its attention to the next situation, they are lost in the storehouse of the memory faculty as deep rooted imprints. These subterranean imprints are neither right and wrong (non-judgemental) but stored exactly in contents at the moment of perception by the waking mind. The seeded impressions lay dormant (figuratively) in the deep plane of the unconscious mind. The surfacing of the hidden memory impressions is set in motion when comparison of new or similar information is brought before the aware mind, needed to form recognition for the individual to respond accordingly to the current situation at hand. The faculty of buddhi (intellect) first makes comparison of the incoming external stimuli to the surfacing past impressions of memory in order to help in the final decision-making. The outcome of the made decision leaves the mind to play out the scenario of the given situation.

In summary, the four internal instruments can be likened to the way physical food particles are ingested, broken down, absorbed, and assimilated by the gastrointestinal digestive organs. Buddhi is the equivalent digestive organ in the mind. It is through the digestive action of buddhi (intelligence) in discrimination (digest), reason (absorb), and decision-making (assimilate) that sensory food images and contents are converted into microscopic thought particles to feed information to the mind. But before the finish thought particle is formed, buddhi signals to the digestive component of memory (smrti) for comparison of past thought particles, so to give the necessary digestive hormones and enzymes to further break down the microscopic thought substance. Once memory processes the food thought particle, it is returned to buddhi to continue the digestive process on the matter of thought. But again, before deciding the final thought form, ego (ahamkara) enters to improvise what condiments (spices) are needed to add flavor and taste to the thought particle so to associate the feel of touch and the sense of being real to the final formation of thought.

Dr. John Cosby

Lower Mind: The Senses and the Physical World

The lower mind has three main components —mind, memory, and ego factor. Together the three components help process the relative information obtained during the waking activities of daily life. The information is then stowed as impressions in the unconscious mind for further use whenever needed. The cycle and recycle of desire, thought, and impressions appear endless in one's life span. Thus, the components of the lower mind interact primarily on a mundane level to fulfill its daily needs in the present and future.

The false ego looks to satisfy its desires by turning its attention toward sensory matters, and thus, relies on the body and senses to meet those needs. Overtime, the false ego has strengthened in getting its needs met. By now, the virtuous qualities of the higher mind in buddhi (pure intelligence) has become weaken and afflicted, and therefore no longer poised in the flow of positivity and spontaneity in thought and action. The higher mind falls victim to the realm of the lower mind, with the ego projecting more possessiveness. The false ego begins to narrow the activities of mind to fulfill its insatiable needs for pleasure and satisfaction of mundane objects. As the ego grows, the mind becomes more identified with the endless search of relative happiness. The strong craves and instincts bind the mind to be subservient to the lower senses and sensory objects. The mind is drawn further away from the core of the higher self toward the absorption into the lower mind.

Mind, Ayurveda & Yoga Psychology

The beauty of the mind is that it has the capacity to be dualistic. That means the human mind stands at the crossroads between the higher mind or buddhi and the lower mind. The mind has the ability to either pursue the spiritual higher mind or be drawn to the senses of the lower self. It can go beyond its conditioned attraction to the pull of the senses which keeps it in bondage to agitation, frustration, fear, and doubt. With the control of mind, one begins to develop the ability to overcome the allure to the lower mind, and instead ascend to the higher mind, and integration of the spiritual personality.

This is beautifully explained in the sixth chapter of the Bhagavad-gita. "One must deliver himself with the help of his mind, and not degrade himself. The mind is the friend of the conditioned soul, and his enemy as well. For him who has conquered the mind, the mind is the best of friends; but for one who has failed to do so his mind will remain the greatest enemy" (6.5-6). "From wherever the mind wanders due to its flickering and unsteady nature, one must certainly withdraw it and bring it back under the control of the Self" (6.26).

The heart of yoga requires constant self-effort to the practices of its many disciplines. One must choose to bring the mind back to the higher self and not let it get swept away by the drama, attraction, and dialogue of the lower self. The many yogic practices are designed to build up strength and resiliency to the mind so that you can raise to the potential of the higher self.

The mastery of mind gives one the ability to remain centered without getting dragged here and there by the undisciplined mind and the appeal of the sensory objects. The basic aim of all yogic disciplines lies in quieting the vibratory thoughts of the mind and mirroring the higher mind in spontaneity and intuitive wisdom.

An After thought

In his interpretation of the *Yoga Vasistha: Utpatti Prakarana* (Vol II Section 88), Sri Swamiji Jyotirmayananda implies the vision of mind is related to the transmission of light, a vibratory state of consciousness. The vibration or movement of thought is a reflection of the mind, and mind is a reflection of the cosmic consciousness. It is the cosmic light that ablest the mind to project vision onto the objects of the outer world. The projected light within the realm of mind shines outward onto the objective world, and the objects there correlate to the vibratory movement of a thought wave. The wave of thought is an aspect of the operative mind, and this allows the mind to give name and form to the entire objective world.

Chapter 2: Samkhya Philosophy

In this chapter we will discuss the principles of Samkhya philosophy to help explain the creation of the human mind and physical characteristics that disperse our universe. The philosophy depicts the universe as dualistic in that there is an emergence between the pure consciousness of Purusha and the primordial creative force of Prakriti (matter) to start the existence of creation and sustenance to all that abides in the universes. This fusion of pure consciousness, the absolute existence of everything, and the creative physical energy of prakriti, together give birth to the infinite layers of consciousness that perpetuates the very existence of everything in the entire universes. The coming together of purusha and prakriti emerges initially the field of cosmic intelligence (Mahat). The role of cosmic intelligence is to project the universal design and creativity to the makeup of the infinitesimal expressions that takes place throughout the universe. The consciousness of cosmos continues to emerge from cosmic intelligence with the field of individual intelligence (buddhi). The separate intelligence of buddhi is the beginning sparks of individuality in the cosmic order of things. Next, the ego-factor (ahamkara) emerges to give a distinctive identity to every individuality. It is at the dynamic junction of individual intelligence, buddhi, and ego (ahamkara) that the existence and development of the human mind comes into the play of consciousness.

Dr. John Cosby

The significance to the ego-factor (ahamkara) shows its imposing influence that directly impact the shape and color to one's perception to gather and produce knowledge and experience the surrounding world.

Samkhya and the Creation of the University

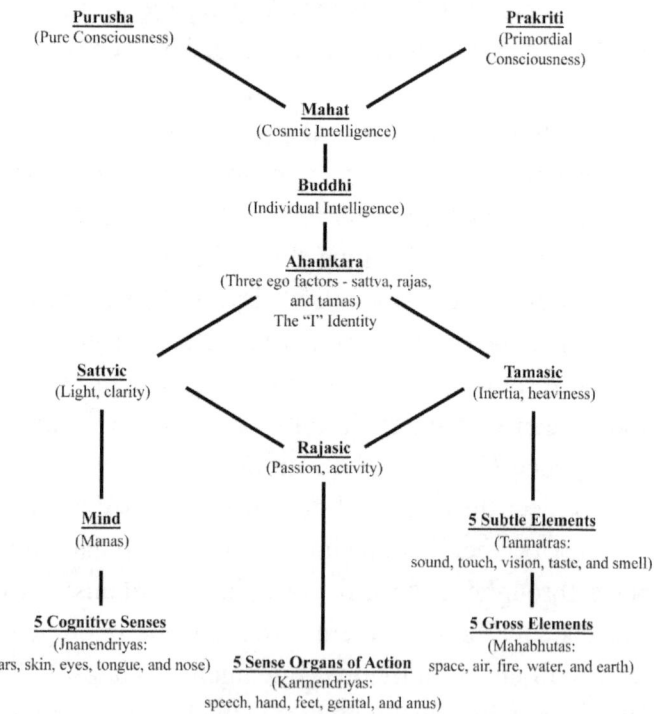

The chart displayed is an illustration of the evolutionary process of Samkhya philosophy, and how it can help us visualize the universal play of consciousness as it pertains to the cosmic players on the worldly stage, and the interconnection to one another.

According to the concepts in Samkhya philosophy,

there are twenty-five elements (or *tattvas*) that comprise the nature of reality to everything around us including ourselves. The pure consciousness of *purusha* underlies the descent of the other twenty-four elements, and thus is the primary essence of all existence. The ensuing twenty-four components role is to manifest themselves into the multitude of forms to be seen and experienced throughout our universe. At the beginning of the creation of all the universes, there is the everlasting pure consciousness of purusha, which lies dormant in its atrributeless state of purity. There is no movement to purusha but just the existence of eternality. It is only aroused to movement by its union with the primordial creative energy of prakriti, which then together stirs the creative forces to start the life forms of the universes. The cosmic evolutionary process continues to enfold through the primordial creatve forces of prakriti, to the emergence of the cosmic mind or *mahat* arises, which the latter is responsible to project, design and define the cosmic waves of intelligence into the innumerable forms as experienced in the past and present worlds, and the continuation into the futuristic existence to everything that takes on a creative form. Next, from the field of cosmic intelligence emerges the droplets of individual intelligence or *buddhi* consciousness. It is at this dynamic cosmic stage of buddhi intelligence that the flow of consciousness emerges into the singular form of intelligence, the beginning of separation from the masses of the cosmos. The individual mind begins to further develop an identity of self (one) through the evolutionary play of the ego or *ahamkara*. The ego factor is comprised of three tendencies or qualities in sattvic (purity and creativity), rajas (activity and passion), and tamas (inertia and heavy). These essential qualities of the gunas blend into distinctive shape and expression into the rise of the immeasurable number of personalities. You can think of the three gunas as the variegated expressions to the numerous snow flakes (unique configuration) that are distinct to other snow flake patterns. Similarily, each of the individual personality is given its distinct characteristics of personalities through the interplay of the inestimable combinations of the three gunas, which offers each individual definition in how it perceives and interrelates within the world.

Now consider purusha, the male energy force. It is

- invisible,
- colorless,
- motionless,
- unchangeable,
- boundless, and
- without qualities,

Purusha shines its brightness into every corner of the universe. It is absolute and unchangeable in its radiating light. It is not separate from light. It *is* light. It underlies the infinitestimal light of every name and form throughout the universe. This glowing light of purusha illuminates the mind in turn to shine its individual reflected light onto the outer objective world so that one can gain knowledge and experience of it. The reflective light of the attentive mind projects its outward movement through the instrumental senses onto the separate and outer objective form. The appearance of objects comes to life only when the mind shines its attention and brightness onto the dualistic form. On the other hand, the mind that is not attentive and lightless to illicit the senses leave it inactive and unattached to the gather of any objective form.

Now consider prakriti, the feminine energy force. It is

- dynamic,
- active,
- visible,
- bounded
- changeable, and
- with qualities,

Prakriti is comparable to the mother's compassionate energy. She gives birth to the countless manifestation of the worlds. The primordial creativity of prakriti flows out of the infinite ocean of purusha to create all matter and energies of the universe (above, below and between). The emergence of prakriti causes the unmanesfested state of that which then becomes the manifested.

The field of consciousness in prakriti remains inactive when the gunas are in equilibrium as a whole. That is the cosmos energy of sattva (purity, transcendental), rajas (activity, passion, mobility), and tamas (inertia, ignorance, delusion) are in balance with each other as one. They remain in a latent state. It is the increase of raja's mobility, onto the other two gunas, that causes disturbance to the equilibrium state of the trigunas that then awaken the primoridial creative energy of prakriti to rise into activity. Prakriti begins to move and merge with purusha to start the creativity and manifestation of everything in the universe that continue to do so at this momemnt.

From prakriti, the first vibrational movement of her primordial creative force evolves into the manifestation of the cosmic mind or mahat. Mahat is the first principle born out of the union between purusha and prakriti. It represents the cosmic mind or intelligence. The intelligence and luminosity of mahat is not a separate force, but it permeates the perpetual cosmic projection of the absolute pure consciousness of purusha and the primordial creative force of prakriti onto everything taking form throughout the universe.

From mahat emerges the manifestation of buddhi or individualized intelligence comes into play on the cosmic stage. The Sanskrit word buddhi is derived from the word *budh*, which literally translates to "awake" or "to know." Buddhi is the beginning expression of individuality in the cosmic play of consciousness.

Buddhi is like a spark of consciousness that has become separated from the overall fire of cosmic consciousness. It is at this stage of creation that pure consciousness is separated into the many lights of individual intelligence. The individual lights (buddhi) develops into the inestimable numbers of created minds since the beginning of human race. The infinite numbers of individual intelligence droplets begin to establish separate identities from one another. Each of the minds being distinct and different from one another.

Although the droplets of individuality appear to be separate and apart from cosmic consciousness, it is united through the omnipresence of purusha and the creativity field of prakriti, but whose appearance of the former is on a microscopic level. It is through the consciousness level of individual intelligence that allow purusha to perceive and experience the many different aspects of the world we live in.

Ahamkara is the individual ego consciousness that evolves from the individual intelligence field of buddhi. The Sanskrit word ahamkara is interpreted to mean ego and self-identification. Aham means "I" and "mine," and kara means "doer," so the compound word literally means "I am the doer." It is in this state of possessive identity that the mind feels separate from others. The state of duality begins to take place.

The ego factor is what gives taste and color to how one perceives, feels, and thinkss of oneself and the relationships of others.

The Three Gunas (Trigunas)

In ahamkara lies the three gunas, which together shape the nature of one's ego. In Sanskrit, the word *guna* means "string" and "single thread." "Tri" simply means "three." Hence, the term trigunas is to be understood. These are the threads that run through everything. Each thing has a certain quality to it, or we might say, each thing has "a certain energy mode." The three gunas (tendencies, qualities, characteristics), are a philosophical and psychological concept developed by Samkhya philosophy.

Sattva is conscious energy. It contains

- Goodness,
- truth,
- purity,
- light,
- happiness,
- peace, and
- tranquility.

Rajas is active energy. It contains

- passion,
- desire,
- activity,
- creativity, and
- motion.

Tamas is inertia energy. It contains

- inertia,
- cloudy,

- slow,
- ignorance,
- inertia,
- confusion, and
- darkness.

Nothing in the universe can escape the influence of the trigunas. It is the very expression of the three gunas' interaction with one another that allows everything to take on unique characteristics both in the physical and mental world. The mind is immensely related to the three gunas, and the inestimable combinations of them are responsible to the development of the many personality traits seen in different individuals.

The essence of ego shapes the individual identity of the person's mind. All three ego-factor play their part into the identity of the individual. For instance, the state of mind demonstrative of the dominating qualities of the sattva ego lies in tranquility and serenity. The sattva ego qualities are exemplified in goodnes, truthfulness, happiness, compassion, effulgent, transparency, peacefulness, and purity. In brightness and clarity, the sattva ego aligns with the above and higher individual intelligence of buddhi consciousness. The sattvic mind is free of impurities, misery and despair. Its only when the predominance qualities of rajas (passion, desire, and cravings) and tamas (inertia, ignorance, and darkness) impact on the tranquil sattvic mind, does it begin to display impure characteristics that can have a negative affect on the mental personality. These negative forces can precipitate into anger, agitation, frustration, anxiety, fear and doubt. The mind then becomes limited with imagination, and thus moves toward the lower senses and bodily consciousness. We will further the discussion on the interchange between the three gunas and mind in the next chapter.

The feminine nature of prakriti continues to progress with its primordial consciousness through the expansion of the sattvic mind with the projection of the five preceptor senses, *jnanendriyas*. The five senses (ears, skin, eyes, tongue, and nose) enable the mind to perceive by hear, touch, see, taste, and smell to make sense of the physical world. Thus, the five senses directly descend from the sattvic mind. From the rajasic ahamkara (activity of ego factor), there emerge the *karmendriyas*, the five organs of action as depicted in the previously outlined illustration. The five organs of action include the mouth, hands, feet, genitals, and anus, which enable the mind to interact with the physical world. Therefore, the organs of action allow one to speak, grasp, move, and direct his or her action within the physical world, whereas the senses of perception help give one's understanding of the world.

The mind is the chief controller of both the cognitive and motor activities. It is the mind that steers the five preceptor senses and motor organs of action. Mind is of a subtler consciousness than the instrumental operatives of jnanendriyas and karmendriyas. Whereas the *indriyas* (senses) connects the mind to the world, its the mind that translates the outer phenomenon into internal knowledge. The indriyas are unaware and unconscious of themselves and their surroundings whereas, the mind is conscious of itself and its surroundings.

For perception to occur, the mind needs to shine its attention on the sensory cognitive organs and gather impulses from the surrounding environment. Thus, the mind becomes active and receptive to the outer physical world when it awakens the sensory organs. The sensory impressions are transmitted via the complex neural pathway to the brain. The mind perceives the incoming impression, processes it, and crystallizes it into a thought wave to give us information and experience. Once the information is processed, the mind responds by relaying a signal or message back to the organs of action. Together, the cognitive sensory organs and organs of action enable the mind to communicate and interact with the material world.

The organs of action are based on how one acts in the world. The five organs of action are all governed by the principle of mobility, which allows one to move and respond to the outer world. Speech expresses movement of our inner thoughts to others through verbalization. Hands move to grasp and hold and exchange external information. Feet enable one to walk in order to get somewhere else in time and space. The reproductive genitalia allow people to procreate and generate new life. The elimination of waste products cleanses the body, and changes the unused material back into the environment.

The Objects of Perceptions (Tanmatras)

The tanmantras are the subtle elements which are objects of the five senses - sound, touch, sight, taste, and smell. The interaction of the tanmatras allows one to sense the objective, tangible and touchable world. It is through the combinations of the tanmatras that arise the gross elements.

The Five Great Elements (Pancha Mahabhuta)

The constituents of physicality found in every part of the material world is comprised of the five gross elements of earth, water, fire, air, and ether, which in turn, gives a particular appearance to that physical form. Internally, the five elements are responsible for the structure and function of every cell, tissue, organ and system operating in the human body. Every object is made up with a predominance of two of the five elements, the other three minor elements impacting less characteristics. These five gross elements are the building blocks of all matter across the dimension of our universe (macrocosm and the microcosm).

Space pervades the entire universe. It is boundless and has no restraints. The inner body's structure (microcosm) and the vast universe (macrocosm) is principally made up of space. The clay pot broken in half does not void the space within the pot. Space underlies the other four elements.

Air represents movement and activity. It is colorless,

Mind, Ayurveda & Yoga Psychology

tasteless, and odorless. It moves the elastic lining of the lungs so we can inhale and exhale. The signal transmitted along the neurological circuitry is primarily moved from one nerve cell to another by the subtle force of air.

Fire is characterized by expansiveness, light, heat, and vision. Man is able to perceive and retrieve the image of the external object through the subtle light of the retina, which lies at the back of the orbital eyeball. The gastric fire is needed to digest foods to be broken down into microscopic size to nourish the infinitesimal cells.

Water is dynamic, liquid, and viscous, and it fills space. It can be restrained (water dam) and contained (reservoir). When water becomes massive in size (floods), it can build up in force and cause damage. The elasticity and moisture permeated in the wall muscles of the heart is necessary to expand and contract to pump blood through it four chambers and circulate the vital components of blood (oxygen) to nourish the entire body. The synovial fluid of the knee joint helps sustain flexibility, prevention of erosion to bone, and safeguards the hinge and ball apparatus of the shoulder against sudden impact.

Earth represents solid, heavy, slow, and static. The skeletal system allows the body to stand erect. The bones and muscle are necessary for locomotion and movement of the body. The brain is encased in the skull to protect it from trauma.

Each of the tanmantras subtle elements of sound,

touch, sight, taste, and smell) corresponds to a particular gross element (i.e., sound to space, touch to air, sight to fire, taste to water, and smell to earth respectively). For example, the vibratory sound corresponds to a wave in space, touch to the air felt against the face, sight needing light or fire to see, and so on. Thus, the tanmatras (subtle elements) enable the mind to perceive the objectivity of the gross elements. In essence, the entire world of matter is made up of the five gross elements.

The following scenario given shows the interplay between the mahabhutas, tanmantras, jnanendriyas, and karmendriyas. For example, the space (mahabhuta) in the sky thunders its roaring sound (tanmatra), which is heard by the ear (jnanendriya). The sound produces thought vibration that allows action in speech (karmendriya) to express the thunderous sound to others.

This is shown in the following chart, the display of each mahabhutas (i.e., gross element of air and space) corresponds to a specific tanmatras (subtle element of sound) which is perceived by a particular cognitive sense (jnanendriya of ears) that correlates to an organ of action (karmendriyas of speech).

Mahabhutas	Tanmantra	Jnanendriyas	Karmendriyas
Space	Sound	Ears	Speech
Air	Touch	Skin	Hand
Fire	Sight	Eyes	Feet
Water	Taste	Tongue	Genital
Earth	Smell	Nose	Anus

In summary, although everything appears to be separate pockets of creation, each unfolding manifestation is actually a continuum of the cosmic consciousness that emerges from the begininingness of purusha to union with prakriti. The pure consciousness of purusha remains unchanged even in its ever-expansion of the universes. The vastness of primordial creativity in prakriti is responsible for all of the living creatures and matter that make up the universe.

Chapter 3: The Three Gunas: Sattva, Rajas, and Tamas

Introduction

In this chapter, I will discuss the three *gunas* in detail; The three gunas (tendencies, qualities, attributes) are a philosophical and psychological concept that orignated from the Veda (Artharva) and later expounded in the Samkhya school of thought in helping explain the working of the human mind. Samkhya explicates the progression of the ego through the concept and interplay of the trigunas to the thinking process of the mind. It is the ego factor of the three gunas that lay importance to the movement of the mind in how it identifies to itself and surroundings. These three gunas are described through the qualities of sattva (purity, honesty, transparency), rajas (activity, passion, materialistic), and tamas (inertia, stable, fixated). They realized how deeply the characteristics of the gunas ingrained on the ego factor of the individual, which in turn, influenced the working of the person's perception, feeling, thought formation, intelligence, reason and comprehension, and resultantly in what manner the individual intermingled on the world stage. It is the qualities of the gunas and the interaction of each on the other that give one insight into the variable and distinctive expressions of the human personality traits, which yoga psychology has used to define and categorized the mental disposition of the person.

The Prevalence of the Gunas

These three gunas are called sattva (harmony), rajas (active), and tamas (inertia). The three gunas are present in all beings and objects but they vary in proportionate amounts to the parts of the whole. It's the qualitative and quantitative changes of each gunas that give the distinctive expression of multiplicity to objects and thoughts. They cannot be separated or removed from the object because they produce the expressive content of the object. They can be increased and decreased through the influence of other external objects and situations. However, it is the aware mind alone that can bring about the increase and decrease of the gunas through the construction of thought content.

The three gunas are constantly interacting with one another because of the expansion of consciousness. The gunas are never in a permanent place in the progression of the relative world as evidenced by the continual changes to the beginning and ending of an object or thought for that matter.

The three gunas appear as a single object. They are not seen as parts to the whole. It is the appearance of the predominant guna characteristics that gives one the perceptive assessment of the labelled object to shine, although all three gunas exist.

The Qualities of the Three Gunas

Sattva	Rajas	Tamas
Purity, honest, truthful, clarity, peaceful, calm, serenity, goodness, calmness, brightness, happiness, intuitive intelligence, and effugence. It is light, luminous, and transcendental in nature.	Passion, activity, energy, impulsive, aggressive, ambitious, motivated, driven, change, desire, and restlessness. Rajas is want of materialistic objects. Its tendency is to cause turbulence in circumstances and thought because of its mobile nature.	Selfish, possessive, gloomy, heavy, dense, resistence, dull, inactive, idle, grounding, cloudy, indolent, ambiguity, and stabilty. Its nature is ignorance and delusion in perception and thought.

The individual can show changeable guna qualities throughout the day depending on the situations, beliefs, concepts, and interaction with others, even though the gunas underlying their conceptive mental personality is basically unchanged. For example, the rajasic person who goes to a place of worship on the sabbath will show sattvic qualities (peaceful) to how they should act during the time spent there, upon leaving the building to go home, and the rest of the day. But on return to the workplace at the stock market the next day, the same person becomes passionate, driven, competitive, aggressive, and charged to handle the fervent stock trades by telephone with others he or she has never met before in person.

The variable expression of the human mind is shaped, shaded, and coated by the fabric layers of the trigunas. The gunas influence the way the mind precieves, feels, and relates to the world around it.

For instance, the perception of the individual mind is influenced and acted out by the predominance of the gunas. Sattvic people will see the entire objective form with accurate precision. They feel as if they are "in a zone," which makes every piece of the object appear as though it's running in slow motion. The raja person tends to oscillate in thoughts, which causes interference in the perception of the image. The restless mind will scan parts of the objective form and not fully see the all-inclusive image. The tamas people tend to be deliberate and slow to action when it comes to surrounding objects. They tend to be resistant to change, and they are fixated in nature. Thus, their perception of the external object can be limited because of their fixation.

Mental Disposition of Sattva, Rajas, and Tamas

It is the predominance of the qualities of the three gunas that defines the individual mental disposition in combination with the two minor gunas, which together reflects how we think and perform with others.

The *predominance of sattva* in people shows

clarity of perception and thought, excellent memory and intelligence, depth of reason and comprehension, and articulate and sincere speech. These people will be truthful and honest in expressing feeling and thought. Their calmness exudes positive energy that draws others to them. They tend to see the positive aspects in relationship and circumstances. The sattvic person possesses a great degree of self-control and never shows agitation and anger. These people tend to be spiritual, inspiring, humble, and self-disciplined in all task that they undertake. They have a natural willingness to help others. They radiate luminosity, joyfulness, and contentment. Others are attracted by their bright aura and personality. The sattvic guna is transcendental in nature.

The *predominance of rajasic* in people tends to involve around worldly affairs. These people are quick learners and swift thinkers. The ragas mind is self-motivated. They are driven to succeed in the material world. They seek material possessions and wealth. They are never satisfied with enough, and they are drawn to achieve and strive to no end for more, which leaves the mind unsatisfied and agitated. They are hardworking. They can be so obsessed with what they are doing that they tend to lack sensitivity in relationships. They can illustrate pride, arrogance, conceit, and greed, and they can be critical, pessimistic, argumentive, competitive, impatient, and envious of others when they are out of balance. The rajasic guna is associated with active energy.

The swift movement of the rajasic mind gives way to impulsive action, rapid thoughts, and indecisiveness, which can devolve into ambiguous feelings, memory decline, self-obsessive ego, poor decision making, opinionated reason, and miscomprehension of the whole picture.

The poise of the *predominance of tamas* tend to relate expressions of compassion, forgiveness, kindness, and love. When tamas is balanced, it reflects the virtuous qualities of a mother's love for her child. These people are wonderful workers, as they bring stability and reliability to the work environment. They tend to be good in relationships because of their caring and loving nature.

The nature force of tamas often slows us down, especially when we need sleep. Sleep is beneficial to healing and restoring energy within the body and mind. It also insulates us from the daily onslaught of activities and quiets the mind for a period of time.

These people's fixated nature is slow, heavy, and resistant to change. They can tend to feel stuck in thoughts and feelings. They can become attached to their feelings to the point of being self-possessive. Life may become routine, tiresome, and tedious with little or no enthusiasm. At the extreme end, one may experience dullness, darkness, lethargy, laziness, apathy, ignorance, greed, and gluttony. They can indulge in criminal activities, heavy alcohol consumption, substance abuse, extreme obesity, and stagnation of mind.

This will conclude the first part of this book in the presentation of the mind.

Part 2: Yoga Psychology

Chapter 4: Yoga Psychology

Introduction

Thus far, the first three chapters have been largely introductory, but now we will begin to get to the heart of the matter. In this chapter we will focus on the most important points of the *Patanjali Yoga Sutra*, an ancient and profound work on the psychology of the mind. The essential theme that runs throughout the book works toward the ultimate goal in life—self-realization. Patanjali gives a number of disciplines to achieve this goal. In them, the individual is able to quiet and then stop all thought waves through one's concerted effort. The intensification of self effort gradually leads to the control of mind. He goes on to say that thought distraction yields agitation, frustration, discomfort, suffering, and misery. The distraction of thought lies in the forms of the *kleshas* (ignorance, ego, attachment, aversion to objects, and fear of holding on to delusion). We will explore the concept of these kleshas and how they harvest anguish and despair, and then in subsequent chapters, we will explore how we go about eradicating suffering and achieving self-realization through the processes of yoga.

Yoga psychology is quite different from the scientific concept of Western psychology in that there is no focus on mental illness. Rather there are purification disciplines to remove impurities and blockages of thought and action so that one can ascend to higher states of consciousness. The focus is on removing the mental afflictions of ignorance, ego, attachment, aversion, and fear (the five kleshas), all of which lead to sorrow and grief. Those are not the forms of mental suffering caused by mental illnesses with a biological component (depression and nervous breakdowns) as given in Western psychology. Yoga psychology is focused on the eradication of the erroneous mental processes so that people can experience the realm of psychological health. Yoga recognizes that the five afflictions are a by-product of the mind. These afflictions are generated by the faulty processes of mental energy, which one can restore these interruption of electric shortages to balance the spiritual personality.

According to Patanjali's yoga sutras, the Sanskrit phrase "Yogas Citta-Vrtti-Nirodhah" literally translates to "the cessation of the fluctuation of all thought waves." We are to eliminate any distraction of thought that may interfere with the attentive mind. In summary, the philosophy of every yoga is geared toward this common end, namely to attain silence and establish a quiet mental space that's absent of thought waves.

Patanjali terms the idea of fluctuation of thought waves as *vritti*. He describes vrittis as waves on the surface of the ocean. Vrittis are mental aberrations that arise from the erroneous formation of thought. They first appear when the mind begins to contract and perceive the outer world. The mind perceives and differentiates the many objective images of the world

Mind, Ayurveda & Yoga Psychology

through the formation of thought waves, and with these, the mind gives definition to the self and its relationship to the outer world. The vrittis formed are then stored. They are either accurate or inaccurate in the gather and digestion of the sensory information. They arise from their storage place (unconscious) to come alive when they are needed to play out the thought impressions on the screen of the mind. In essence, the thought wave of every new and retrieved image creates another ripple movement on the surface of the mind. One can only imagine the large number of thought waves generated in a lifetime.

The strength of vrittis is related to the degree of pleasure and pain. Pleasure is movement toward desirable objects, and pain to the avoidance of undesirable object. Pleasure and pain have the same capacity toward either attraction or distraction. Vrittis are in themselves expressive replications of every desire played out by the mind. In essence, the obtainment of pleasurable and painful objects is what leads the mind to be distracted and obsessed with the desirable object. The preoccupied and interrupted mind is pulled by the strong attraction of the senses to the desires of the objective world. The mind becomes enfeebled and sacrifices the space of stillness and quiet for the gain of imagery thought activity (vritti).

Dr. John Cosby

Kleshas: Afflictions of the Mind

The Sanskrit word *klesha* translate literally to "poison and contaminate." Patanjali describes the mental afflictions or kleshas as the basis of all human pain, suffering, and misery in the world. These mental afflictions are divided into five main catergories.

- avidya (ignorance or a lack of knowledge),
- asmita (ego and pride of self),
- raga (attachment),
- dvesha (aversion and hatred), and
- abhinivesha (clinging to life or the fear of death).

The Sanskrit word *avidya* literally means ignorance and delusion. Patanjali goes on to say that ignorance is the foremost agents amongst the kleshas responsible for every affliction of the mind. Avidya or ignorance is the deepest impression of the mental afflictions and thus underlies the rise to the other four afflictions. The other kleshas or mental afflictions exist secondary to avidya. Avidya and the subsequent four kleshas give rise to defective patterns of thought that are played out on the world stage. In essence, ignorance veils the mind from seeing life with accuracy and purity. The indefiniteness of perceptions and thoughts stain one's view of realty.

Out of ignorance rises the second klesha, which is called *asmita* (false ego). The ego's essential characteristic is possessiveness and ownership. This false identity precipitates into the very fabric of one's personality. The ego expands the space of mind, and the individual often thinks, "*I am important, I know better, this is mine*, and *that's yours.*" The mental personality is threaded with the fabric of the ego.

The deceiving ego covers the eye of mind with its own agenda. The subjective mind is saddled by the imposing ego and moves in a direction of want to benefit itself. The intellect of the mind becomes subservient to the needs of the selfish ego.

Asmita gives rise to the third and fourth kleshas, raga and dvesha the afflictions of attachment and hatred respectively. Raga is the attraction of mind to the pleasure received from objects and circumstances. The feeling of pleasure surrounding the desired object adds intensity to the attachment. The repeated attachments become seeded deeper in the unconscious mind. The unconscious mind is enticed to chase after the desirable pleasure, as there never appears to be enough. There is never an end to the acquisition of money, possession, fame, lust, power, etc. The increase of raga creates an illusory reality of attachment, which fails to bring permanent happiness.

The fourth klesha, dvesha, is characteristic of aversion, repulsion, rage, and other dislikes that arise in response to negative experiences (e.g., having one's life threatened, a breech in security, humiliation, one's happiness taken away, and other painful circumstances).

The feeling of discontentment makes people avoid uncomfortable experiences. They distance themselves from others and situations. These negative sensations, if left unresolved, precipitate into displays of irrational emotions, whether knowingly or unknowingly.

The afflictions of attachment (raga) and aversion (dvesha) are complementary to the other. They cause one to diverge from one's nature way. The person's feelings become polarized to the extremes—pleasure and pain, love and hate, happiness and sadness, highs and lows, likes and dislikes, and joy and sorrow. The divergent mind is encumbered with emotion of opposites and mentally live in a space of dither thoughts.

Holding onto the embodiment of attachment and aversion leads the mind to the fifth klesha, abhinivesa (fear of death and clinging to life). These false notions of life are deeply rooted in the collective unconscious of the masses, whose strong grip direct fear to the active mind, often times to act habitually. The mind becomes troubled by the uncomfortable feeling of separation rising even though it may not even realize the undercurrent of it. Most fend off the ideas of separation (e.g., losing one's job and livelihood, facing the death of a family member who has a serious disease, and the possibility of identity theft.) with irrational thinking. The mind cultivates defense mechanisms to protect itself against the painful feeling of separation. The instinctive buffer zones are setup, and these tend to be harmful too. After all, most enemies are illusory. Our guarded behavioral patterns are put into place, and we act upon them. Our protective mechanism softens the feeling of losing something that's too valuable. The anticipated idea of losing our physical body and all of

Mind, Ayurveda & Yoga Psychology

our possessions can give way to fear, confusion, and depression. The thought of never seeing a loved one again can cause extreme turmoil. The loss of personal space and the prospect of someone else controlling us can bring on apprehension of others. The idea of losing our self and what we stand for can create tremendous fear within our psyches. We have invested so much in building up the sense of the ego self. With these irrational beliefs about loss, we may start to believe that they could actually become real.

The experience of the plane of objects, senses, and thoughts goes down deep into the unconscious, where it is stored. There is no gap between the present experience and impression, all of which is stored in the unconscious mind. Nothing is lost between the subtle transition of the actual experience and the past impression stored into the unconscious. Everything is preserved down to the smallest detail.

When you see and taste an apple for the first time, you gain actual knowledge of the apple. The perception and impression of the apple by the active mind is immediately stored in the unconscious in the form of memory. Thus, the impression is stored in the memory bank of the unconscious. The impression is retrieved from the memory bank when the apple is again perceived by sight of the waking mind. The mind recognizes the color and shape of the apple, and taste of it. Thus, the object and the act of knowledge are distinguishable but not separate from each other.

The kleshas lie deep within the depth of the

unconscious mind. There they lay dormant, ready to come alive and respond to a particular situation at hand. These hidden kleshas or latent impressions are known as *samskaras.* Samskaras resemble seeds soiled into the deep ground of the unconscious. There they begin to sprout upward to the subtler subconscious's fertile soil to further their growth to maturity. In the subconscious these afflictions change into the form of subtle desires that lies just beneath the conscious mind, ready to use. These subtle desires are known as *vasanas,* and if allowed to go unchanged, they spring to the conscious mind in the form of thought waves. The thought wave form and act in accordance to the imposing impression of the vasana. It is at the conscious level that the ripened vasanas bear their fruit in relation to the external world. Thus, the afflicted impression or kleshas stored in the unconscious rise to the subconscious to formulate subtle desires into thought waves, giving rise to acts in the form of hatred, jealousy, self-centeredness, greed, anger, selfishness, attachment, fear, sadness, obsession, infatuation, illusion, and other contaminated thinking, which in turn filters into the bloodstream of one's personality.

The kleshas are difficult to remove from the unconscious plane. For one, repeated patterns of thought waves are dug deeper into the grooves of the recorded device of the mind. Two, the distracted mind is mostly unaware of the impressionable to kleshas, and thus left to act on patterns of instinct and impulse, which does not typically change how one thinks. To complicate

Mind, Ayurveda & Yoga Psychology

matters, these afflicted thoughts are tightly wrapped in electrically charged feeling, which makes them more difficult to separate without the awareness of one's prejudice of them. Thus, these unresolved feelings rise to color and shape one's thought and actions. The unaware mind is overridden by the negative afflictions of the kleshas, which deprives the former of cogent reason and intellect.

In summary, the cause of all misery and suffering originates from avidya and plays out in the cyclic stages of afflictions by the mind as illustrated in the following chart. Once the person goes through each of the afflictions, the cycle restarts over and over until the chain of the afflictions is broken by the practices of yoga disciplines. Swamiji Joytirmayananda beautifully lectures often on the topic of the kleshas (Yoga Research Foundation in Miami, Florida).

Kelshas: The Cyclic Afflictions of the Mind

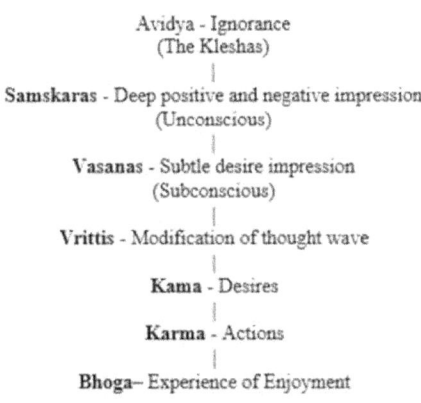

Dr. John Cosby

Karma

The law of karma is defined as the sum of a person's action, whether good and bad, in this lifetime and past lives, which has a strong influence in deciding one's outcome in present and future existences. When one thinks, speaks, and acts, it intiates a force that will react in accordance to the original force of action. It is the equivalent to one of Issac Newton's law. "For every action there must be an equal and opposite reaction." In essence, karma governs the universal principle of cause and effect, which determines how one will think and act in future circumstances. The reverse mental force can be changed or modified to the intitial force of action on how one alters their thinking pattern and behavior.

Th persistence of self effort can be applied to change one's thinking to modify the action in *avidya*, which begins the cycle of afflictions played out by the mind as per the law of karma. The repetitive action of ignorance recycles the negative impression back into the unconscious plane in the form of *samskara*. As mentioned earlier, the latent impressions are awakened by an external stimuli presented to the mind, which then arises in a corresponding subtle desire or *vasana*. In the subconscious mind, these manifest as *vrittis*, modified thought waves. These modified thought waves play to the needs of the desirable pleasures (*kama*) in the external that turns into action (*karma*) which then give the experience of the enjoyable object (*bhoga*) sought by the wants of the individual. Another important player to consider is the false ego, which orchestrates sentiments, which build into intense passion. Together, the pieces of the cycle of afflictions coerce the unaware mind and urge it to seek satisfaction through repeated desirable objects, which means it only recycles the afflictions again and again.

Later we will further discuss samskara and its effect on how the mind forms thoughts and actions in relation to both the present and future circumstances (karma). As stated earlier, samskara is related to the expression of deep-rooted impressions. These deep-rooted impressions begin to take form when the subjective mind directs its attention to the perception of a particular object. The act of perceiving the object is divided into three stages. The first stage is *the perceiver*, who focuses light onto the object. The second stage is *the act of perceiving* the illuminated objective form and its characteristics. The third stage is apprehending *the form of the perceived object* by the subjective mind. Together, the mind considers the objective form separate of oneself. The information of the object is processed by the mind. The subjective mind then transcribes the perceived object into a particular thought wave, which is then crystallized into a related content of an impression and stored in the memory bank of the unconscious.

These hidden impressions, the planted seeds of karma, create ever deeper grooves as a result of the cycle of afflictions. The cycle of the impressions strengthens over time, which then produces an even greater influence on the operative working of the mind.

Dr. John Cosby

These cyclic habits become automatic and instinctual in force that subliminally overtake the distracted mind and its performance in real-time reactions to external situations.

In themselves, samskaras are neither right nor wrong. They are merely expressions of stored impressions that are brought to the surface (figuratively speaking) in response to external stimuli. The mind does not distinguish between positive and negative action. Rather it simply forwards the related content, which can then influence its operation.

The feelings of anger, hate, neediness, jealousy, obsessive, distrust, fear, and precocious behavior are strong negative samskaras. The greater the intensity, the deeper the grooves in the unconscious record. These hidden emotional markings tend to stand in the way of the mind's natural response to certain circumstances. The negative samskasras blind the vision of mind and therefore hamper one's ability to think. If the negative impressions go undetected, it can cause troublesome effects on the operative process of perception, intellect, reason, and comprehension of interrelationships and life experiences.

The sequential movement of psychological pain experienced by the mind is illustrated in the following chart in a shorter form by Swami Jyotirmayananda:

The Chain of Psychological Pain

Ignorance
(erronance thoughts)

Egoism
(false self identity)

Subconscious and Unconscious Planes
(subtle desires and impression)

Object of Thought
(attachment and aversion)

Acts of Desires
(pleasure and pain)

Agitation
(unresolved attainment of desire)

Delusion
(fabricate the impression)

The cycle of psychological pain begins when the mind inaccurately perceives a presented external object or situation. The erroneous thought (*ignorance*) of the external object becomes believable primarily because of self importance by the *ego*, which creates a false self-identify (ownership). The outer impression is then brought inward to the mind and simultaneously seeded in the soil (content unchanged) of the deep *unconscious* plane. The mind is left to act on the immediate impression on which way it decides. The impression brought to the fertile ground of the unconscious, overtime, germinates to maturity and begins to sprous (subtle desires) upward into the *subconscious* mind. While lying in the subconscious, the subtle desire (vasanas) remain virtually hidden just below the conscious mind until it is awakened by some external stimuli. When awakened, the subtle desire ascends to the conscious mind and helps form an *object of thought* in regard to the current external stimuli. The object of thought is left for the mind to respond to the stimuli at hand. The perception of the thought content takes on the twofold action of either: want (attachment) or avoidance (aversion). The duality of attachment and aversion intensifies into the feeling of pleasure and pain (*acts of desires*) respectively, which in turn gives a sense of realism to the object of thought. In essence, the pursuit of the duality of want or avoidance of the material image is never permanent gained but always temporary in nature. Thus, the transcient satisfaction of the object of thought is never completely obtainable. The unresolved attainment of the *(external) object of desire* causes one to experience agitation and frustration. The failed attempts to permanently attain the desirable object causes the mind to become even more disenchanted (*delusional*), which causes one to deceitfully sidestep the painful experience by fabricating a false impression to evade the illusory object.

Chapter 5: Ashtanga Yoga: The Eightfold Path of Yoga

> "Manojaya eva mahajayah."
> Translation: "Conquest of mind
> is the greatest victory."

Introduction

In the beginning of this chapter, I will provide a brief dialogue of the eight limb of ashtanga yoga found in the ancient text of the Patanjali sutras. In the next chapter a detailed of them (asana, pranayama, etc) will be given. In essence, the consummation of the eight limbs centers on the purification of mental impurities through a series of philosophical and practical steps. The practices of the eight limb gradually remove the distracted thoughts that seems to fill up the mind. The elimination of thought content advances the person to be in control of their mind. The mind free of impurities advances the mind to become a basis of subtler sentiments, intellect and reason which they provide a different dimension to the emergence of an inner (higher) being. Consequently, the inner light of knowledge begins to grow in intuitive intellect which spontaneously unifies into self realization, the ultimate goal of ashtaanga yoga.

The systematic order of the eight limb begins with the ability to restraint the individual needs, advancement of society values, steadiness of body through yogic posture, control of one's breath, withdrawal of sensory objects, advancement to single-minded concentration that develops into uninterrupted meditation, and finally, the achieving of enlightenment.

The eight limbs are categorized as

1. *yama* (restraint/code of conduct),
2. *niyama* (ethical/religious observances),
3. *asana* (postures),
4. *pranayama* (control of breath),
5. *pratyahara* (withdrawal of senses),
6. *dharana* (concentration),
7. *dhyana* (meditation), and
8. *samadhi* (super-consciousness).

But before these first two steps (yama and niyama) can be undertaken, one needs aspiration to begin the journey. Aspiration is the inner belief that there is a higher supreme being that underlies all existence in the world. Only then can one start the practice of yama and niyama toward achieving the eight limb. Both work simultaneously to make one aware of the self in relation to oneself, others and society.

These two practices are followed by the third limb, which focuses on body postures called asana. If properly done, these allow the body to experience quietness and relaxation. The practice of asana strengthens both body and mind through steady and disciplined poses. The resiliency and elasticity of the body renovates the electrical circuitry of the nervous system. Other benefits include the entire network of muscle, tendon, skin, and bone to reach maximum pliability and flexibilty to the body.

The steady and comfortable poses help remove tension buildups in the physical, emotional, and mental planes of the individual. Whereas the gym workouts stimulate the body to relax, asanas offers composure and quietness of the bodily components so that they can be free of tension, stress, and edginess. This creates a pacify and positive effect on the mind. Without agitation and distraction, the mind feels lighter and vibrant in perception and content of thought.

The mastery of asanas prepares one to undertake the subsequent stage of pranayama (breath exercises) followed by pratyahara (withdrawal of senses), dharana (concentration), dhyana (meditation), and finally, samadhi (super-consciousness), all in the effort to accomplish the eight limbs of ashtanga yoga.

The Eightfold Limb of Ashtanga Yoga

The First Limb—Yama

Yama is the first of eight limbs of ashtanga yoga. It is the most external of the eight practice. It is the beginning stage of gaining control over the mind towards the final goal of self realization, knowing the true nature of oneself.

Yama consists of five restraints/code of conducts that are universal and not limited to any one group, religion, culture, and society. These include *ahimsa* (nonviolence), *satya* (truthfulness), *asteya* (not taking the possessions of others), *brahmacharya* (abstinence of negative thought/celibacy), and *aparigraha* (abstinence of greed). These are often seen as a collection of ethical vows to what people should not do.

Although at first it appears the restraints deal with internal workings, the code of conduct is external so that one can start controlling his or her actions without harming others. The emphasis is on eliminating injurious deeds through avoiding wrongful acts of violence, lies, stealing, sexual indulgences, and covetousness.

It begins only when the mind develops a strong will, which will help restrain one's action for the benefit of the self and society. Yama constitutes the universal code of conducts, and these vows run contrary to the impure acts of killing, injury, stealing, lying, hoarding, indulgence, and selfishness. It is through self-discipline and right action that one removes injurious thoughts and deeds.

Then one is left to express positive values of compassion, peace, and kindness to others, uphold goodness, honesty, and truthfulness in society.

The Five Restaints—Code of Conducts of Yama

Ahimsa is the first directive of yama. The term is coined from the two words *"a"* and *"himsa"*, which literally mean to avoid any harm or injury to all living creatures and nature. Nonviolence goes beyond harm

Mind, Ayurveda & Yoga Psychology

of the physical body alone. Damaging thoughts project violence in expression of hatred, anger, jealousy, greed, and selfishness. One should restrain him or herself from falsehood too—untrue conversation, hurtful speech, and negative thoughts about others. The person who lives with truth expresses honesty in thought, speech, and action, which helps to sublimate the spread of violence in society.

The power of speech is more destructive than physical injury, and negative thought more so than vocal speech. "The pen is mightier than the sword" literally means words are more powerful than an army. Words should be spoken wisely. One should consider how one thinks before speaking.

Vedanta placed greater emphasis on the restraint of nonviolence (ahimsa) in comparison to the other yamas. It recognized the fact that the underlying thread throughout every yama is related to the principle of ahimsa. Thus, the rectification to any of yamas is always handled first with ahimsa.

Satya is the second yama that is the buildup of ahimsa through honesty and sincerity. It constitutes truthfulness in every action. One should always give truth in thought, sweetness in word, and be good and do good in action. Truth in thought is the transfer of spoken knowledge that benefits everyone. Satya refrains the intent of falsehood in thought, deception in word, and injury in action. The expression in dishonest thought underlies violence toward others. Honesty is the abstinence from any violence. Speech should not

Dr. John Cosby

be deceptive or misleading because it can then cause *himsa* (harm) to others.

Astreya is the third directive of yama. It is abstinence from stealing from another. The very act of stealing from another is based on one's greed and voraciousness. It lacks the control over the senses (selfishness). Even thinking about stealing causes pain, hurt, and sorrow to another even though the act has not been committed physically. The desire for someone else's possessions is governed by the law of karma, and thus, you will reap the injurious deeds you commit against another.

Brahmacharya is the fourth directive of yama. Brahmacharya is related to satya in purity of thought, word and deed. In essence, it strongly refrains the idea of lust from entry and control of the mind. It is abstinence of avariciousness in sexuality, both physical and mental infatuation of lustful thoughts. It is one of the strongest forms of bondage to break in comparison to others.

Vedanta teaches one to practice the complete cessation of sexual impulses and action, that is necessary to reach the final goal in self-realization. As long as the sexual instinct is superlative, will it interfere with self-realization.

Tantra proposed control over the sexual thrust by implementing secret techniques to prevent the downward release of sexual energy. Instead it teaches one how to hold and harness sexual fluid (creative life energy) in order to move upward from the *muladhara* to the *sahasara* chakra and experience higher consciousness.

One who controls the release of sexual fluids preserves and invigorates the forces of ojas and prana, to rise vertical to the sahasara chakra.

Aparigraha is the fifth directive of yama. It urges one to avoid being covetous and greedy. The disciplined mind recognizes the need to reduce the desire to accumulate wealth beyond what is necessary or what is required to sustain comfort in one's life. It requires self-discipline to stop the acquisition and hoarding of material objects, which reveals the underlie motivations of greed and gluttony. The desire to acquire possessions and wealth makes it difficult for one to live at ease and instead causes more resistance in the mind.

Second Limb—Niyama

Niyama is the second of the eight limbs of ashtanga yoga. The five directives of niyama are designed to purify body and mind (*sauca*), satisfaction and contentment (*santosa*), strengthen the will through austerity (*tapas*), listen and reflect on the higher knowledge of the sacred scriptures (*swadhyaya*) and gurus, and finally, to help one completely surrender the individual self to a higher being (*Isvara-pradnidhana*).

The Five Ethical—Religious Observances of Niyama

Sauca is the first directive of niyama. It is purity of the physical body and thought/mind. The physical body is given proper nourishment to strengthen and optimize the bodily functions and systems. Organic foods, proper exercise, and proper rest builds up strength to bodily constituents. Clean clothes, sufficient air in the room, and the absorption of sun's rays helps to establish a healthy body.

On a deeper psychological level, the cultivation of positive thoughts purifies the processes of the mind. Positive thoughts help to cleanse the mind much like one cleanses the home. The effect of positive thoughts spreads to purify the inner heart which yields expression of generosity, compassion, and kindness.

The purification of the mind sublimates thoughts of negative feelings of anger, greed, jealousy, conceit, and aggression. Negative thoughts make the mind impure, distracted, and leaves to the waste of mental energy.

Santosa is the second directive of niyama. It is the abstinence of desire. The contentment and happiness of the mind does not search outside for external fulfillment and enjoyment. The contented mind no longer looks for transient gratification but enjoys what is at hand.

Contentment and satisfaction occurs when there is want of nothing more than what is necessary to fulfill the basic needs of body and mind. It is the realization that the accumulation of unfulfilled desires does not bring happiness. Rather it is the realization that true happiness of the self is abstinence of unnecessary wants for worldly objects.

The mind filled with the sattvic characteristics of happiness, joy, and contentment sublimates the passionate tendency of rajasic to seek more material wealth and tamasic's heavy grip on not letting go of one's possessions and selfishness.

Tapas is the third directive of niyama. It is designed to make the physical body strong and help one develop the mind in order to refine concentration so that one can work toward growth in spiritual personality. Concentrated effort helps make the mind stronger in attention even when exposed to opposite sentiments, such as joy and sadness, adversity and prosperity, happiness and unhappiness, loss and gain, and pleasure and pain.

Austerity in speech should be joyous in manner and not a burden on one's psyche. It expresses no harm to another with crude words. *Satyam Vada, Priyam, Vada, Na Vada Satyam Apriyam* literal translates as "Speak the truth, but do not speak that which hurts others."

Svadhyaya is the fourth directive of niyama, which includes the study of sacred scriptires (Vedas, Upanishads, Puranas, Bhagavad Gita, Bible), the repetition of mantras (Om, Gayatri, Om Namah Shivaya, Hare Krishna, Soham), and the reciting of holy hymns, such as the Guru Gita. The reciting and reading of the svadhyaya strengthens the mind to sustain concentration, reflect, and meditate to gain insight into these sacred texts.

Isvara-pradnidhana is the fifth and last directive of niyama. It is the reminder to surrender one's words, thoughts, and actions to the omnipresence of the divine self. On a psychological level, it is the release of one's ego in order to selflessly serve the higher. The service of surrender helps free obstacles of the mind in negative thoughts and substitute virtuous qualities of goodness, honesty and righteousness.

Yama and Niyama are complementary to each other. They do not work alone. Yama and Niyama both share the common factor of restraining the external mind in how the individual acts in accordance to the needs of society. Yama uses the code of conduct to begin the movement of restraints on the mind, whereas niyama is based on behavioral observances to society. Yama imposes self-discipline so that one can know what not to do. It is concerned with how one acts appropriately in relation to society. The yamas and niyama pass through one another to better the individual and values of society.

The Third Limb—Asana

Asana is the third limb of ashtanga yoga. The literal meaning of asanas is *seat*. The reference of asana here is meant to signal the many postures that make up the physical practice of yoga. The posture movements of asana should be done in a smooth, relax, and comfortable manner. One should hold each posture steady over a period of time. The great sage Patanjali perfectly capsulates the picture and position of asanas in the yogic sutra "Sthira Sukham Asanam," which translates to "A pose that is steady and comfortable is called asana."

Mind, Ayurveda & Yoga Psychology

Asana is a systemic series of postures that integrate sound structure and function to improve the body and maintain a healthy frame of mind. These postures have been shown to give physical, psychological, and spiritual benefits. Physically, the asanas mechanical approach eases and stretches joints, muscle, bone, and organs in their natural shape and form. Mentally, each asana builds steady and calm awareness of the inner and spontaneous flow movement of thought. An awareness of gentle breath helps to ease thoughts and feelings, which correspondingly relieves bodily and mental tension during the position of each posture. In turn, one softly breathes with his or her lungs to increase the oxygen supply, which in turn nourishes the peripheral organs, glands, muscles, and joints. The slow and gentle intake of full breaths helps one relax the body's muscles and joints, and the movement on exhale helps the person remove deoxygenated, acidic waste and buildup of physical tension. The set movements of opposing postures (flexion and extension) with alternating inhale and exhale rhythm helps to move awareness to that particular musculoskeletal system being worked on. Another benefit of steady asana and conscious breathing is that they soothe and revitalize the nervous system and make them stronger and more resilient against the daily stresses.

When repeated postures are perfected does tense feelings, distress, and thoughts of frustration wane to help one return to a calm state of mind. A composed body without disturbance allows the mind to gently focus on the task at hand, and in turn, one can also sit for longer periods of silence in meditation.

The Fourth Limb—Pranayama

Pranayama is the Sanskrit word taken from the root derivatives of prana (life energy force) and ayama (mastery or control). The purpose of pranayama is to regulate the flow of oxygen and prana through breathing exercises. Over time one becomes aware of the spontaneous rhythm of breath. Prana is the subtle vital life force that gives life to all creation. It is the energetic force that sustains life from the moment the fetus comes alive to the time of death. Without prana there is no life. When speaking of prana we do not mean oxygen or air, both of which requires the life force of prana to come alive.

Physically practicing pranayama is meant to help one develop the natural rhythmic flow of inhale and exhale during one's daily activities. One can increase the lungs' capacity to hold more fresh oxygen and prana (higher retention) in order to maximize the functions of body and mind. But more than just accomplishing a physical feat of regulating breathing, it aims to arrest the intensify feelings and thoughts that circulate endlessly.

> "Tasmin Sati Shwas Prashwasayor
> Gati Vichchedah Pranayamah."
> —Raja Yoga 11–49.

Translation: "having perfected Asana or posture, and when the movements of inhalation and exhalation of breath is mastered, is it called Pranayama."

Prana and mind are interconnected. One can discover the middle between prana and mind lies in the movement of breath. Breath has a direct effect on both prana and mind. An awareness of the mind can train the lungs to take in and retain more oxygen and prana, which then has a positive effect on the psychophysiological systems. On a physical level, not only the intake of prana and oxygen is beneficial but also the expellation of bodily toxins and waste. In a psychological sense, coordinated breathing on the smooth flow of inhale and exhale help to release negative residual emotions and thoughts. The buildup of negative thoughts and emotions causes waste in energy to retard the optimal processes of the body and mind. The regulated and deep movement of breath supplies higher prana not only to the body but causes expansion in thoughts of lightness, calmness, clarity, serenity, strengthen and invigoration of mind.

The great sages acknowledged the correspondence of subtle channels that run parallel to the circuitry of the nervous system. These subtle channels are called *nadis*. The nadis support the flow and circulation of subtle prana in order to energize the subtler bodies (gunas) and the seven psychic centers of the chakras. The charged life forces of prana flow simultaneously along the subtle nadi channels and the circuitry routes to the nervous system. The flow of prana and nadis are inseparable. The pranavahi nadis (channels of the nadis) carry the prana life energy to the different parts of the body, which represent the life forces of the universe but on a microscopic level.

There are more than seventy-two thousand nadis throughout the body. The larger seven chakras (major nadis) or psyche centers (muladhara, swadhistana, manipura, anahata, visuddhi, ajna, and sahasrara) have greater influence on the personality traits of the physical and mental bodies. The nadis connect the life sources of the cosmos in the form of prana through the nervous system of the physical body.

In diminished states of prana, there is an increase of impurities attributed to shallow rhythmic breathing, wrong choices in foods, negative thinking, unhealthy habits and addictions, a buildup of stresses, and unresolved emotional exhaustion. The yogis acknowledge the regular practice of pranayama is needed to purify the nadis and allow the full flow of pranic energy to rejuvenate the entire nervous system and function of the human body.

The Fifth Limb—Pratyahara

Pratyahara is the fifth of the eight limbs of ashtanga yoga. Pratyahara is the withdrawal of the senses of perception (indriyas), to focus the internalization of mind from being drawn to the external world.

Pratyahara is not limited to the sensory organs of perception but also the sublimation of the interplay of possessive thoughts and dialogued in the mind. Pratyahara is the alleviating of the dominance of the senses craving sensation of desirable objects. On a more profound level, it is the practice of breaking mental habits to strengthen the mind to perceive the grosser perceptions to a subtler feeling, intellect, and reason of one's wholesome inner being.

The mind relies on the indriyas to satisfy its taste for contents of the external. When the desire becomes too strong does the mind become subservient to the needs of the lower senses. The unattentive mind moves from its inner core of strength and will, thus gives its power to the outer (transient) world. Figuratively, the mind is held captive by the lower senses. The mind is led to believe it cannot exist alone without the senses.

Pratyahara concludes the external limbs of ashtanga yoga.

The Sixth Limb—Dharana

Dharana is the first of three internal disciplines followed by dhyana (meditation) and samadhi (super-consciousness). The last three of the eight limb are essentially internal practices to silent the mind to achieve self realization. The beginning five of the eight limb (yama, niyama, asana, pranayama, pratyahara) were practiced to bring the externalization of the mind towards the internal self.

Dharana is derived from the root derivative of *dhri*, which literally means holding. In a yogic sense, dharana is the hold of single-minded concentration on any particular object. The discipline of dharana is to control the flow of mental distraction to the development of a single flow in thought.

Dharana is the inward movement of an idea, thought, and object being used to harness and sharpen the focus of the mind. The progression of dharana is dependent of intention and discipline in order to develop a strong concentrated mind.

The object that the person chooses allows for a magnetic attraction to raise the mind to hold a greater concentrated state of attention. In turn, the compelling force of the object helps one develop mindfulness concentration.

Tratakam is a concentrative meditation practice that requires focusing (with open eyes) on a particular external object. For example, people frequently use the flame of a candle to develop concentration. At first, the watery eyes may blink excessively, but with practice, one is able to hold his or her attention on the flame.

The Seventh Limb—Dhyana

Dhyana is the seventh limb of ashtanga yoga. Dhyana is the result of repeated effort that brings one-pointed concentration (dharana) to the practice of meditation where the mind continues to focus without interruption. The continuity of intensify concentration helps to remove

Mind, Ayurveda & Yoga Psychology

mental distraction which earlier had interefere with the process of mind to sit for uninterrupted meditation. The practice of medtitation (dhyana) further involves the mind to focus with continuity onto a single point of attraction and hold the attention on it, without any disturbance in thought. This is different than dharana, which the flow of thought is funneled into a single concentrated effort on an image. In dhyana, the object of attention is the mindfulness flow onto a desire object, image of diety, or the sound of a mantra. The chosen object of focus should be relevant to a higher vibration for easier absorption onto the object. Its purpose is to center one's hold and absorption onto the form of the object to anchor the mind without interruption of thoughts. At this stage of deep meditation there is complete absorption between the object and the mind. In essence, the person becomes the object without any separation between the two (perceiver and perceived). Dhyana moves the seer (subjective) so that he or she is absorbed into the seen (objective). The subjective is absorbed completely into the true form (svarupa) of the objective.

The Eight Limb—Samadhi (Superconsciousness)

Samadhi is the eighth and final limb of ashtanga yoga. The progression of intense concentration and uninterrupted meditation clears the way for the mind to go beyond the movement of thought and be completely absorbed into the form of the object, as one. In this sate of mind, the advance perceiver emerges intuitively into the object, with no separation of thought and action. There is a true and pure unity of perception and the object of perception. The subject is no longer limited to the time process of past and future. One just experiences the existence of being in the present.

Conclusion

To illustrate the eight limbs of ashtanga yoga, we can imagine an allegorical journey one must take to reach the state of enlightenment. To begin the journey, the driver must be grounded with the necessary knowledge to follow the progressive steps in order to finish the expedition, which is to reach the palace of the heavenly king. The driver has prepared the journey before hand by practicing yama and niyama to control his and her self restraint and observance, which gives one the proper guidance and alertness so to stay straight on course to the palace. Again, before starting the long journey, the practice of asanas is implemented to tone and strengthen the muscles of the horses so to be able to push the chariot for the full distance of the expedition. The fourth step on the path, pranayama, is practiced to regulate the horses' breathing capacity to give vital life energies to sustain the will of the horses to keep a smooth and steady pace. The fifth step is pratyahara, which limits the distractions of the horses by placing blinders to the sides of the eyes (senses) so that they can hold their attention straight forward to act together as one. The feet, which are the locomotive organ, are held at a trotting pace by the driver (mind) who controlls the movement of the horses by holding the stirrups. The sixth step, dharana (concentration), allows both the horse and driver to stay straight ahead without wandering off to the side of the road. The effort of concentration by the driver and horses make for synchronicity to one another. The seventh step is dhyana, which establishes a relationship of horse and driver to become uninterrupted in focus of the pursuit to finish the long journey. The accomplishment of intense concentration achieved through uninterrupted meditation by the driver has quietly enfolded the journey to reach the final destination, namely the heavenly king (Samadhi). Upon entry into the grounds of the heavenly palace, one enters into total silence, joy, and bliss. The finish journey to the heavenly king give way to waves of contentment and serenity. The mental journey has been finally completed, and the driver (self) has fulfilled his or her true dharma or duty with selfless devotion to becoming one with the heavenly king in the royal palace, thus reaching the state of enlightenment.

Chapter 6: Asana and Pranayama: The Science of Postures and Breath

> When the breath wanders, the mind is unsteady, but when the breath is still, so the mind is still.
> —Hatha Yoga Pradipika, fifteenth century

Although asanas and pranayama were discussed earlier in chapter 5 as the third and fourth limb within ashtanga yoga, this chapter will disscuss in depth that of asana and pranayama.

Asana

The positioning of asana pose also involves breathing, which serves as a precursor to the practices of pranayama. The yogic practice of asanas is considered the sisterhood of ayurveda. It has been practiced for thousands of years in the East. Today yoga is widely practiced for different reasons. It has been shown to reduce stress, calm the mind, improve focus, stretch the body and used for a form of exercise. Socially, it helps people reduce the toxicity of modern living in tight quarters. Whatever the reason for doing yoga, the individual procures positive benefits as a result of the different styles of asanas.

For the purposes of our discussion on the asana systems, the postures illustrated in this book will essentially be hatha yoga. Hatha yoga and its variations are the most common yogic postures practiced throughout the world. Asanas combine different postures with conscious breathing to maximize the relaxation of the body and mind. Holding postures for extended periods of time reduces distraction and tension within the body and helps one regain his or her natural movement. The goal of asana is to hold each posture in a comfortable and steady position.

The regular practice of asanas tones muscle, invigorates organs, increase the suppleness of bodily parts, and helps to relieve resistance in the body. It betters communication between the physical and mental bodies, and it helps the mind improve concentration and composure. It also quietens the mind so that one can sit longer in meditation sessions. The hold of the postures builds up isometric strength to the body, and bring stillness and levelness to the mind.

There have been thousands of studies to date on the stress reduction associated with the regular practice of yoga. Yoga modulates a posivitive affect on the receptive nerve endings of the body and adjusts the automatic nervous system and endocrine glands' responses to negative stimuli and stress. Yoga has helped revise mental perception so that people can readily adapt to current stressful situations. Countless laboratories findings have shown us the medical benefits of yoga. It can lower blood pressure, regulate heart and breathing rates, reduce excessive cortisone secretion, and decrease episodes of migraines, anxiety, panic attacks, and depression.

Dr. John Cosby

In conjunction with yoga, breathing is imperative to quieting the mind and nervous system. Breathe directly effects emotion and feeling, whether positive or negative. The impurities expressed in feeling have an imaginary effect on thought and vision, to the make of how things seem to appear. The negativity in thought has a damaging effect on the nervous system and function of brain, which are responsible for relaying and translating information between each cell. Cancer is the disoriented communication between cells. It increases aggression and the destruction of other cells. Thus, asanas and breath are powerful purifying methods to cleanse the constituents of body and mind.

Pranayana

Pranayama relates to doing breathing exercises. These breathing exercises have a significant effect on the rhythmic flow on inhalation and exhalation. One who controls the breath is able to control the body and mind. On a deeper level, it is practice to prepare one to enter more deeply into meditation. Pranayana, the science of breath, is taken from the derivative root words *prana*, meaning "vital life force," and *ayama*, meaning "to control." Pranayama techniques are done to regulate breath control and increase pranic energy throughout the body.

Prana is the subtlest life force, whose energy lies beneath the creative movement of the world around us.

Mind, Ayurveda & Yoga Psychology

Its life-giving force sustains the existence of everything, whether animate or inanimate.

We should not misunderstand prana, or we should not equate it with the air we breathe. It is not the air that makes up our atmosphere. Rather it is the very life energy of the molecule of air. The currents of prana flow with energetic nourishment between and through the air molecules. Prana can stand on its own, whereas even air is dependent on the life energy of prana to exist. Prana charges the air and oxygen to come alive in order to feed the subtle constituents of the physical body and brain.

The human body needs a constant supply of prana to sustain health. Health and prana are interconnected. The opposite premise holds true as well. The deteriorating medical condition of the person with severe respiratory distress (despite the fact that he or she is put on a ventilator) moves closer to death. Even with a sufficient flow of oxygen, the ventilator fails to prevent the inevitable loss of life. The mechanical respiration system is programmed to supply the correct percentage of oxygen needed to sustain life, but it is still unable to hold off death or bring back life. The life-giving force of prana gives and sustains life, and without prana, there is no life.

Prakriti is the primordial energy that creates and permeates the entire realm of the human race. Prana serves prakruti and gives life to the human body and subtle mind. Physically, prana is the life source that moves essential life energies in order to sustain the cells, tissues, organs, and systems of the body. Psychologically, prana moves sattva, rajas, and tamas gunas to shape and mold the personality aspects of the mind. Prana is the essential energy force that breathes life into all the workings of the physical and psychological aspects of the human. Without pranam there is no human activity.

> "Tasmin Sati Shwasa Prashwasayor
> Gati Vichchedah Pranayamah."

> Translation: "After the steadiness
> of asana or posture, the control
> of ingoing and outgoing of
> breath is called Pranayama."

The ancient yogis recognized that the vital life force of prana could be controlled by the regulation of breath. Breathing is related to the reflective wave movement of prana. The wave movement of prana is the microscopic reflection of the cosmic prana. The balance of the breath rhythm on inhaling and exhaling allows one to replicate the natural wave movement of the cosmic prana. To control the wave movement of prana is to allow the expansion of the mind so that it can go beyond its limitation and experience higher vibration of consciousness.

The integrity of the senses and working mind are dependent on the directive wave movement of prana.

The mind and prana are interdependent. Breathing is the medium that connects the prana energy force to

Mind, Ayurveda & Yoga Psychology

the individual mind. The control of either mind or prana leads to the control of the other. The control of prana expands the boundary of mind so that one can become creative, imaginative, and intuitive. The mind that is calm without distraction in thought makes the breath flow with spontaneity and smoothness. The conscious awareness of steady breathing and mind gives rise to the expression of joy, harmony, serenity, and happiness. On the other hand, irregular breath that is shallow and rapid can instigate expressions in worry, fear, confusion, headache, and muscle tension in the body. The mind then displays the negative expression of anger, passion, jealousy, envy, and hatred. Negative thoughts decrease the vital energy of prana, which weakens health and opens people up to illness.

Prana is the force that moves the mind. It enables the mind to flow in a given direction and space. It is the progressive movement of the individual mind into the objective world to gather data and comprehension of it. Prana moves the mind toward the senses to retrieve outer information and bring it inward so thought and knowledge can be formed.

Prana and the mind cannot be separated. Together, they act as one force to the directional movement of a singular thought. This can be illustrated by the structure of a dam that allows a certain amount of water to pass through it. The right amount of force from the rushing water has to be calculated with precision. Otherwise, too much water will pass through the dam opening and rush forth with a destructive force to the valley below. The force that moves the water forward can be compared to the life force of prana and the watery movement of the mind. Although they appear to be of two separate workings, in actuality they are one and the same. To control the movement of water, one has to control its force at the top of the dam. Similarly, to control the movement of mind, one has to control the higher force of prana.

Practice of Pranayama

Pranayama is an effective yogic practice designed to build up prana energy. By the continual practice of pranayama, one increases the retention of life force to manifest a high energetic charge for the constituents of mind.

The basis of pranayama is to establish the continual flow of prana. The easiest way to absorb and extract prana for the body is through the regulation of breath. Organic foods, appropriate exercise, and positive thinking are other ways to absorb prana.

Pranayama should not be mistaken as the intermittent attempt of someone slowing down his or her breathing. Although slowing the intake of breaths helps to exercise the lungs, it has a limited effect on the pranic absorption of practicing pranayama. Pranayama is more than just the act of slowing and stopping the breath.

Pranayama is the conscious practice to control breath with a purpose. It is to regulate the rate and rhythm of breath—oxygen and prana—to nourish, soothe, balance, and invigorate the nerve plexus (nadis) and network (nadi channels). The greater the amount of prana and oxygen retained, the more soundly the nerve cells effectively operates and transmit signals to the automatic and sympathetic systems. Thus, prana is associated with the capacity of the nervous system, the intermediary faculty between the outer and the subtle mind, that relies on high levels of the former to function optimally.

Breath Mechanism

I will illustrate two points to explain the basic breathing mechanism of the body. First, the accurate way to inhale is through the nostrils. The nasal passageway is paramount to the purification of air molecules, and it prevents other microscopic particles from entering the throat and lungs. The walls of the nasal passageway are lined with cilia, tiny hair-like structures, and mucus membranes. The cilia and mucus membranes are there to catch foreign particles, which are then prevented from going any farther into the respiratory passageway.

Nasal breathing traps most microscopic particle, airborne germs (viruses), and dust from entering the pulmonary compartments (esophagus, trachea, bronchia, and lungs). Nasal breathing is the primary line of defense in the respiratory process (along with the skin, which breathes too). Breathing through the nasal passageway allows the body's natural immunity

Dr. John Cosby

(nose, throat, and tonsils) to fend off a major percentage of unwanted particles.

Unabashed mouth breathing allows particles to infiltrate the mouth and throat. The mouth is not equipped to stop microscopic airborne particles from entering the respiratory system. An open mouth increases the possibility of undesirable airborne particles to colonize the body, which makes one susceptible to pharyngitis, strep throat, bronchitis, exasperated asthma, among other respiratory illnesses.

Rhythmic movement of nasal breathing is paramount to the intake of maximum oxygen molecules and the expulsion of wasted gases. A reduction in oxygen (through an obstruction of the nasal passage) and the buildup of airborne impurities can cause fatigue and headaches in the body as well as restless thoughts in the mind.

The full breath on inhalation uses the entire lung capacity by expanding the lungs outward at the chest area, and the diaphragm to stretch downward to the navel area. The complete breath uses the entire diaphragm to fill the lungs with the maximum supply of oxygen. The diaphragm muscle plays an important part in the expansion and contraction of the lungs. The breathing exercise causes the diaphragm to move in a natural flow with no resistance. The movement of breath should be smooth, easy, and comfortable. The idea is one should not force breath whether inhaling or exhaling. The natural flow of a full breath obtains the maximum benefits with minimum effort and waste of energy.

When exhaling, the diaphragm should contract at the navel point upward to the inferior border of the ribs and further up to the upper lung area. The contracting diaphragm carries a vibratory force that comes in contact with the liver, spleen, stomach, intestines, pancreas, heart, and lungs. These vibratory expansive and contractive movements of the diaphragm massage and stimulate the circulation of blood to these organs and adjacent bodily parts. Moreover, the full movement of the diaphragm discharges impure toxic gases (carbon dioxide and nitrogen) and other airborne waste products out from the respiratory system.

In the western hemisphere, most people unconsciously inhale to a third or half of their full lungs capacity and thus limit the quality and quantity of oxygen molecules. In today's climate of space, the majority of the world's population live in the confines of big cities where the quality of air is sometimes not enough to fulfill the needs of the physical body. The lower percentage of the quality of oxygen adversely affects the entire body and mind over a long period of time. The inadequately oxygenated mind and body coupled with stress may cause one to experience increasing fatigue, depleted energy, heaviness, aches, and pains. The body responds to this lack of oxygen by breathing faster, shallower, and with shorter spurts to compensate the spiraling demands of the mind. The depleted mind slowly dissipates into greater disturbance and rapid thought processes.

The old saying "Take a deep breath" illustrates the importance of using the movement of breath in moments of irritation, anger, frustration, confusion, and restlessness. The partial intake of breaths limits the demands of oxygen for the entire functions of the body. Thus, the middle and lower lobes of the lungs are not being used at a time when they are needed as well.

Complete Breath

The complete breath exercise is comparable to the way nature intended us to breathe. Natural breathing uses minimal effort and energy and the maximum efficiency of the lungs' capacity. The principle of complete breath is to use all three lobes of the lungs during inhalation. The right lung is comprised of the upper, middle, and lower lobe. The left lung consists of the upper and middle lobe only. The left lower lobe is displaced by the placement of the heart. The complete breath fills the entire bilateral lobes and maximizes the levels of oxygen and prana.

Conscious breath with awareness gives attention to the subtle sensation of air movement through the nose, throat and trachea. One can then listen to the expansion and contraction of lungs and the movement of the diaphragm. The mechanism of breathing should be done in a synchronous flow.

One should state the practice of complete breath

control in the lotus position or sitting comfortably in a chair with his or her back straight and feet flat on the floor. Observe any discomfort in the body, and release the disturbing sensation with soft and gentle breathing to the area. Feel the spontaneous flow of breath in and out several times to relax the body and mind. Then begin to focus the mind on the flow of breath through the opens of the nasal down the passageway of the throat and upper chest area, filling completely the upper, middle, and lower lobes of the lungs. Simultaneously, there is a gentle movement to the expansion of the chest wall, lungs, and diaphragm. One should not jerk or force the breath in any way.

On completing the inhalation cycle, there is a subtle space that begins on its own and ends just after inhalation and before exhalation. Quietly sense this space with closed eyes, and then witness the narrow space that takes place between inhalation and exhalation.

On exhalation, feel the flow of breath without resistance move up the lobes of the lungs, trachea, esophagus, and throat and out through the nasal passageway.

The complete breath exercise can be practiced anytime. Awareness of the breath is necessary to settle down the respiratory movements and establish a natural and spontaneous rhythm that offers relaxation and calmness to the mind. The following is a breakdown of the lotus position. You must sit on the floor cross-legged with the back erect. However, if you cannot sit on the floor in the lotus position, then you can instead sit in a chair with your back erect in the same way.

- Sit in padmasana (lotus position) or in chair with back erect and comfortable.
- Relax the body muscles, and release the heaviness of thought.
- Feel the body and mind move effortlessly.
- Begin by inhaling in a smooth, rhythmic flow through the nasal passageway.
- Feel the flow of breath into the throat and down the esophagus and trachea.
- With awareness, follow the breath flow into both lungs.
- The flow of breath to the upper part of lung softly raises the upper ribs and simultaneously pushes the diaphragm downward and upper chest wall forward.
- The fill of the upper lobe allows the flow of oxygen to enter the middle and lower lobes. Observe the slow expansion of the lungs outward, the downward motion of the diaphragm, and the abdomen wall's movement forward.
- Filling the three lobes with air simultaneously pushes the chest cavity, ribs, and intercostals muscles to expand outward in one downward motion.
- Filling the three lobes of the lung should be in a continuous and smooth motion. It should be one movement without jerkiness.

- Once inhalation is finished, hold the breath for one to two seconds, and become aware of a subtle and inner space without resistance.
- Now exhale the flow of breath from the lower lobes slowly with the diaphragm muscle moving upward and inward from the abdomen wall.
- Upward exhalation continues to empty the lobes of air, which causes the diaphragm to push slightly upward. Gently contract and push inward the lower and middle ribs, intercostals muscles and chest wall.
- Then slowly exhale the breath from the upper lobes with the diaphragm moving more upward and the upper ribs and chest wall more inward.
- Again, the breath should be exhaled with evenness and no resistance.
- You should perform this exercise two to three times. Do not force or strain any movement.
- The complete breath should be done with a relaxing and gentle awareness. Once practiced a number of times, you can do it while walking and standing. Please avoid driving and other dangerous activities while you are practicing the complete breath movement.

Nadi Sodhana—Yogic Cadence with Breath

Nadi shodhana is derived from the Sanskrit words *nadi*, meaning channel, and *shodhana*, meaning cleansing and purifying. Together, the purification of the nadis or astral pranic centers allow for the flow of vital life forces to the nerve plexuses throughout the body.

Nadi shodhana uses an alternate nostril breathing technique to purify and cleanse the pranic channels so that there is an unobstructed flow of the life energies to the central and peripheral nervous system. It helps to increase the concentrated index of prana passing through nostril breathing and the expansion movement of the lungs to the distant cells.

The natural flow of alternate breathing brings equilibrium to the two hemispheres of the brain. The two halves of the brain can be aroused and fed prana and oxygen by the use of alternate rhythm of breath. The control of breath through the left nostril stimulates the right hemisphere or the abstract and creative aspects to the working of the brain. Likewise, the regulating of the right nostril breathing invigorates the left hemisphere, which commands the tangible skills of language, logic, and verbalization. Synchronizing the left and right hemispheres opens the bilateral channels of the brain to operate as one, thus increasese states of awareness, clarity, spontaneity, creativity, and intuitive wisdom.

The flow of prana through the channels of the mind brings on a subtle awareness, and it also allows for the removal of blockages of negativity from the channels of the mind. The increase of positive pranic force overcomes the daily strain of fatigue and exhaustion, distress, tension, and agitation.

At first, the practice of nadi sodhana can be

Mind, Ayurveda & Yoga Psychology

cumbersome since one must use different fingers to alternate the flow of breath between the nostrils. But with practice and concentration, the use of the pads of your thumb, ring, and little fingers become automatic. One of the first benefits people notice after this exercise is the feeling of calmness and the relaxation that comes to body and mind.

- Sit comfortably in padmasana or in chair with back erect and feet planted shoulder length apart.
- Shut the eyes, and quiet the entire body.
- Silence feelings and thoughts.
- Practice the complete yogic breath several times.
- Start by inhaling and exhaling the breath on cadence of the ratio of one to one for one minute.
- Close the right nostril with right thumb pad and simultaneously inhale through the left nostril on the cadence of four.
- After completing inhalation, close the left nostril with the right ring finger.
- With both nostrils closed, hold the breath for the cadence of sixteen.
- Release the pressure of the right thumb on the right nostril, and exhale through the same nostril with the count of eight.
- Then inhale through the right nostril with the cadence of four.
- At the end of inhalation, close the right nostril with the right thumb.

- With both nostrils closed, hold the breath for a count of sixteen.
- Open the left nostril by releasing the right ring finger.
- Exhale through the left nostril with the cadence of eight.
- Then inhale through the left nostril with the cadence of four.
- At the end of inhalation, close the left nostril with the right ring finger.
- Close both nostrils on a count of sixteen.

This is one round of nadi sodhana. Repeat the practice five to ten times when you first begin. If you feel light-headed or dizzy, stop right away because you may be forcing the cycle rhythm. It is best to start with a yoga instructor.

The inhale is on the cadence of four. You should hold your breath on the cadence of sixteen. And the exhale is on the count of eight. The inhale and exhale should be smooth and even without strain or forceful movement. If the cadence of 4-16-8 is too difficult, you can begin with the cadence of 2-8-4.

Corpse Breath

In the corpse breath pose, you lie your back on the floor and face upward toward the ceiling. The length of the body is vertical from head to toe. The arms and legs are spread slightly outward from the body to create symmetry.

Mind, Ayurveda & Yoga Psychology

The hands are palm down and limp. You begin the pose by observing the inhale, and then you exhale breath to every part across the body. Light attention is given to any bodily areas of tightness, stiffness, and shifting movement. The mind can gently direct breath to the areas of tension in order to dissipate the uneasy feeling. After listening to your body, the muscles, joints, and skeletal system should be become relaxed and flatten to the floor.

- Gently inhale and exhale the breath through the nostrils several times.
- Begin the exercise by placing full attention on the rise of the inhale and the fall of the exhale in the abdomen area.
- Feel any tension in the abdomen, and relax it with soft and rhythmic breath.
- Next, slowly direct the attention to the toes and release any discomfort with soothing breathe for approximately ten seconds or more.
- Now move your attention upward to the feet, ankles, knees, and legs. Each body part lets go of its tension with soothing and rhythmic breath.
- Move the attention and breath to the fingers, hands, wrists, elbows, and arms area.
- To release any tension to these areas, breathe smoothly and with awareness on inhalation and exhalation.
- Now direct soft and rhythmic breath to the neck area and unto the head to free any deep and distracting thoughts.

- On finishing the exercise, return your attention and breath to the heart area.
- Begin to meditate, and feel the warmth, lightness, joy, and expansion of the heart.
- Many practice this exercise for approximately fifteen to twenty minutes, or some will fall into a sound sleep, which also helps to ease tension and stress.
- The corpse breath posture is a naturally rejuvenating position that helps repair the circuitry of the nerves and body. It offers beneficial effects even though it appears simple and easy. It is wonderful for relieving the body of stress, which restores quietness within the mind.
- Deep breathing used with rhythmic movement is a wonderful conjunction that can be implemented with conventional medical treatments of depression, anxiety, panic attacks, mental fatigue, insomnia, incessant chatter of thoughts, and other stress-related disorders. Meditation, yoga, tai chi, biofeedback, transformational counseling, and limited pharmaceutical intervention are wonderful (though mainstream) complimentary treatments for mental diseases.

The practice of the previously outlined breathing exercises will have immediate benefits if done on a daily basis over a period of time. The regulated breathing pattern will bring calmness to thoughts and emotions, generate more energy, and help one feel more relaxed. The benefits to the controll of our breathing, if done before meditation, will carry over to give us deeper meditation practices. The synchronized rhythm can be practice during the day when you walk to and from of home and while you are running errands. This will help you establish a mental atmosphere of tranquility.

Chapter 7: Thoughtless Meditation

Achintaiva param dhyanam.
—Sri Shankcaracharya

Translation: "To be thoughtless is the highest form of meditation."

Yogas Citta-Vrtti-Nirodhah.
—Patanjali Yoga Sutras

Translation: "Yoga is the cessation of the thinking mind."

Introduction

In this chapter we will talk about meditation. Thus far we have discussed the external limbs of ashtanga yoga (yama, niyama, asana, pranayama, and pratyahara). Meditation comprises the second internal practice of astanga yoga (dharana, dhyana, and samadhi). All three stages of the latter are just different levels of meditation. The first stage, dharana, is when one begins to hold inner awareness, the second stage, dhyana, is when one begins to hold inner awareness on a more continuous basis without disturbance, and the third stage, samadhi, is when one is able to perfectly hold inner awareness at all times.

We will talk about two basic types of meditation—silent meditation and mantra meditation. The scope of meditation is to have the person meditating with no distraction to reach thoughtless moments or rather *gaps* of space between thoughts. Both forms of meditation have the same goal of holding the inner awareness without vibratory thoughts.

Thoughtless Meditation

The ancient rishis' timeless teaching on yoga and meditation arose to guide the human mind so that one could go deeply inward and experience one's true self. The rishis themselves experienced the power of intuitive meditation and gleaned the vastness and depth of the infinite wonders of the worlds. They experienced the inner absolute silence underlying everything in the universe. This absolute silence is the primeval energy force or pure consciousness, which is responsible for the cosmological manifestation of every creature and circumstance.

Through intuitive wisdom, the sages witnessed the absolute and eternal silence, and from it comes the enfolding of perpetual consciousness. It had no qualitative attributes, and it was without limitation. It is forever unfolding in all direction. Absolute silence lies in everything above, below, and in between.

They realized the absolute silence rested in the gap between thoughts, and it permeated the entire universe. In relationship to thought, they recognized the gap to have infinite potential energy waiting to rise in expression as seen in the thought movement into the sound of speech. The gap space is absence of motion until it vibrates into sound frequency and manifests the absolute silence in name and form into the material world. The vibration of sound is the first of the five tanmantra (subtle elements to rise out of ahamkara tamasika). Thus, the wave of sound creates the beginning aspects of the physical world. Sound gives expression to the other four tanmantra in the order of touch (air), vision (fire), taste (water), and smell (earth). Each of the tanmantra (subtle preceptors) helps the mind to perceive the multiplicity to the outer physical world.

The following illustration shows the gap space that gives rise to the process of thought wave and particle and how they descend back into the absolute silence.

Thought is both Wave Form and Particle

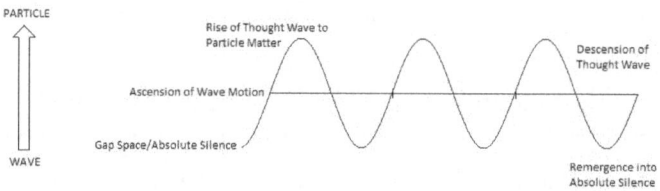

Absolute Silence

The previous illustration shows the potential energy field at the gap space between each thought wave. It appears as a single movement of thought in the formation of a wave into a particle, and then the particle

Mind, Ayurveda & Yoga Psychology

(matter) converts back into a wave form (energy) and remerges into the silence gap space respectively.

Sound emerges from the gap space to give a qualitative expression—in this case, the emergence of thought wave to rise. The ascending thought wave goes on to crystallize the energy form of the wave into a subtle particle matter. The use of wave and particle gives spatial and mobility configuration to thought, which gives the objective appearance to be real. The appearance of wave and particle are not separate but exist as one unit in the processing formation of thought. Neither of the elements are constructed or destroyed but merely changed from energy to matter and vice versa.

The gap space between thought lacks the ego. There is neither ego nor qualities in the gap space but only the potential of silence. It is the plane of pure consciousness in the gap space that allows one to express spontaneous creativity, lucidity in thought, and intuitive intelligence.

Tamasika ahamkara, the heaviest of the gunas, begins to crystallize the thought wave into a subtle particle (matter) of thought.

To illustrate the subtle thought activity, we can consider a quite pond with a view of a magnificent mountaintop overshadowing the valley beneath. Sprouted throughout the valley fields are colorful and majestic flowers. The panoramic view is astonishing and picturesque. It is a beautiful sunny and warm day. A young boy comes down to the edge of the pond on a lazy summer day. He looks at the pond's surface and sees no movement. The stillness of the water gives the

Dr. John Cosby

boy a playful smirk. He is able to see the clear bottom of the pond from the edge of it. The boy playfully bends over to pick up a pebble near his right foot. He then angles his throw and aims the pebble toward the middle of the pond. He throws the pebble straight up, and it falls downward and strikes the center surface of the pond. Simultaneously, a big splash at the surface sprays water away from the pebble. The pebble begins to sink downward and spirals to the bottom of the pond. The pebble just below the surface of the pond causes large bubbles to form. As the pebble continues its descent, the size of the bubbles becomes smaller until the pebble hits the bottom of the pond. The boy notices the bottom of the pond has no more arising bubbles. Only the still pebble lies there. He takes in the quietness of the pond and thinks about playing the game again. He picks up another pebble and starts the scene again.

The pond represents the spectrum of the mind, which holds the movement of thought. The boy is likened to the action of the mind. The mind gives choices to what action to take toward any situation or not. The boy decides to start up the activity by throwing the pebble into the pond. The top surface to the pond represents the physical world where most of us interact on the world stage. The splash of the pebble in the pond causes the start of wave movements. The larger ripple movement is representative of the gross thought movement on the pond of the mind. These wave movements are the surface thoughts we entertain throughout the day to day activities of one's life. The downward movement of the pebble is characteristic of the descent of the grossest to subtlest of thought waves. The descent of subtlest thought waves can be compared to the decreased sizes of the bubbles. The smallest bubbles are characteristic of thought waves moving toward the least resistance. The cessation of any movement of the pebble at the bottom of the pond is similar to the mind having no thought activity or resistance but rather absolute silence.

The daily verbal dialogue and background noise is illustrated by the big splash and the bubbles at the top surface of the pond. Most people throughout the day work at the top level of the pond. They may not even be aware of the ongoing dialogue that has taken place. It's as if the chatter has always been there and part of daily life. The mantra is a tool of transforming the mind to help convert one's heavy thoughts to lighter and subtle ones with less resistance and more mental energy.

The use of a sound (mantra) can be used to move the mind to progress deeper into the pond of meditation to experience subtler consciousness until there is no thought but complete silence. Allegorically, think about the pebble descending with less bubbles and resistance to where it finally settles peacefully at the bottom of the pond.

The rishis recognized the intimate relationship between sound and mind. Language uses sound to pronounce syllables and words to enable one to express thoughts. Most people use their minds to speak what they are thinking at the gross level. Words and thoughts can have different influences on how the mind perceives the spoken image. The image of a cobra passing by your feet sends the body into a flight mode, and the mind reacts with the hissing thought of fear and fright. The wide smile of an infant with big bright eyes cuddled in your arms gives rise to feelings of love, warmth, and tenderness. Thoughts are used to give particular language patterns an expression for a certain effect.

The potential for attaining higher levels of consciousness lies in tapping into the gap between thought waves and the stillness of the pond. The subtle vibratory sound of mantra is a tool that can assist one in disengaging from gross thought activity.

The Art and Science of Meditation

The sages long knew that the absolute silence in the gap space was the underlying consciousness found in the makeup of the universe. The potential to attain higher states of consciousness lay in tapping into the gap space between thought waves. The sages knew one could achieve this by delving deeply into meditation to reach that space of absolute silence. Deep meditation without resistance and thought activity could bring you to experience the unqualified silence. One could bring the gain experience of silence from meditation back into one's daily life activity. The tapping into the space through regular meditation could also allow one to transparent to higher states of consciousness.

Sit for Mantra Meditation

To begin the practice of mantra meditation, one should sit cross-legged in the padmasana (the lotus) position or sit with the back straight upward against a hard chair or wall. The spine must be straight to allow the pranic energy to fully circulate through the vertical patterns of the body. Sitting for meditation in a slouched position blocks the energy from moving circumvent and upward. Before beginning mantra meditation, one should relax the large and small muscles of the body (feet, ankles, knees, legs, buttocks, abdomen muscles, lungs and chest, hand, elbows, arms, shoulders, neck, face, tongue and mouth, forehead, and eyes). The mantra should be silently recited with slow cadence, and focus to the space between the eyebrows. This technique has the capacity to raise the pranic energy in a vertical line to the intuitive third eye. As you meditate inwardly, listen to the rhythm of the breath by watching the movement of the chest expand on inhale and then contract on exhale. The inhale and exhale movements should be done through the nose breath and not through the mouth. The doing of breath work before meditation will soften and quiet the body and allow the mind to experience faster depth of the mantra with less resistance of thought and more space in silence.

Regular meditation will teach you to sit quietly and motionless for longer periods of time. Watch to keep your back straight and vertical with no residual tension to the muscle and joints especially the neck area.

This will help the body become more relaxed and free up oxygenated energy to better circulate through the various areas of the body, which in turn will calm the mind and help you achieve deeper meditation.

As you experience deeper levels of stillness, you will begin to lose your awareness of the body, which will free the mind of images and chatter. The expansive stillness brings on less effort of the person meditating.

The sound of the mantra must be done effortlessly and with joy. The intent to practice meditation is to master the sound of the mantra. It's much like training the mind to learn an important skill. The choice of the mantra should be given by one who knows the mystic formula of the combination of the root letter(s) that vibrate a higher frequency in your mind. Then you can generate a spiritual and magnetic effect in your consciousness. One should develop internal quietness to listen to the subtle sound of the mantra. If the awareness of the mantra becomes distant or stops, softly repeat the mantra effortlessly with a relaxed mind to bring it back to the space between the eyebrows without forcing or mentally holding onto it. The repetition of the mantra should not be mechanical or done with little interest.

After meditation, give yourself time to relax by lying down comfortably for several minutes, and remain quiet in the peaceful state. You should distance yourself from any outer interference. This is the period to reflect on the stillness or gain some insight in your life.

Mantra Yoga

Mantra yoga is one of many yoga practices to help fabric and blossom your spiritual personality. The Sanskrit word *mantra* has two roots. The root *man* is associated with the mind, and *tra* means protect. The literal meaning is to "protect one from the attraction of worldly thought processes and to establish the mind in deep concentration."

Mantra is the process of translating active thinking into deep concentration. It is the cessation of fluctuating thought to help one focus on an object, which leads into uninterrupted meditation.

The ancients used mantras. They used an internal object so that the mind could descend into deeper concentration. Mantra uses the sound to assimilate the vibration of the image. The objective is to develop awareness of the mantra sound rather than give any word form or meaning to the image. The mantra sound has no preconceived idea, concept, and definitive meaning and thus cannot be place into language form. Thus, the mind uses the sound of the mantra to experience the true nature of the objective form rather than any association of it.

Mantra yoga is based on the science of sound. It is derived from the mystic formula of specific sounds. It uses an exact and scientific root letter structure. The mantra sounds were derived from precise configurations of root letters taken from the fifty alphabetic letters of Sanskrit, the purest and oldest phonetic language used today. The letter(s) arrangement of the mantra is not related to any physical form or thought-language pattern but rather to its intrinsic eternal sound. The high frequency of sound waves of the mantra has a powerful vibratory influence on the mind.

The single syllable sound that formulates the mantra is called *biji* or seed sound. Biji is the essence force that lays embedded in the mantra. The *bija* is the divine form within the mantra. It is the abode of divine consciousness. It is through repetition of the bija seed of the mantra that invocations of the divine energy can be used to advance human consciousness toward intuitive knowledge and wisdom. The power of the biji sound has the ability to transform the physical, emotion, and spiritual planes.

In the spoken language, sound vibrates into the expression of letters, syllables, and words to produce meaning in speech. Speech is the gross form of the subtle sound. The mind gives rise to thoughts and produces speech to verbally exchange one's ideas and feelings in outer relationships.

The Practice of Mantra Meditation

The purpose of meditation is to cease or slow the activity of thought that draws our attention outward. The continuum of restless thoughts seems to fill the quiet space of our minds. In meditation, there arises gentle awareness to calm down the restless images that fill the mind. The regular practice of mantra sound allows the mind to experience greater quiet, which then naturally slows down the person so that he or she can let go of the passing thoughts. In the progression of meditation, insightfulness develops to the point of a witness state to watching these passing thoughts as separate units and not the customary stringing of them. The background noise of thought eventually fades to the quiescence sound of the mantra. The quieting effect of the mantra draws the attention inward so that one can experience silence.

Repetition of mantras should be done with no effort or forced attention on it. The sound of the mantra is repeated softly and effortlessly. The flow of the repeating mantra moves naturally. There is no forced cadence to the mantra. There is gentle awareness of the mantra without affixing to it. The spontaneous effort gives way to quiescence and transparency of mind. The space of mind widens for a greater awareness.

If thoughts arise during meditation and diverts attention away from the mantra, one should gently place awareness back on the mantra. The awareness of the mantra lightly replaces the focus of the mind back on it. There is never any resistance to movement between mantra and thought.

Breath is the bridge between the mind and the mantra. Breath can reflect the state of the mind. Breath that is deep, slow, and rhythmic allows the individual to experience ease, contentment, and joy of mind. Breath that is shallow, irregular, and superficial casts the mind into nervousness, irritation, and rapid thoughts.

Dr. John Cosby

Breath Is Meditation

In meditation, mantra and breath are synergistic to one another. Controlled breath allows awareness of the mantra to flow evenly and naturally. The movement of the mantra becomes smooth with no resistance and jerkiness. The vibratory sound wave becomes subtle, and their influence gives an even cadence to the rate and rhythm of breath. The smooth cadence in rate and rhythm reciprocates the movement of the mantra sound so that it becomes even more subtle and concentrated. The breath and mantra sound becomes intertwined in singular movement. Yogis have known that to slow the cadence of breath in meditation means to remove any resistance in body and allow the mind to expand its space in order to experience widen states of consciousness.

The practice of meditation should be done with clear and precise intention and dedication. The individual's intention is most important to the development of the mantra so that one can go deeper in concentration and subtlety. Clear intentions acquiesce the mind so that one is able to sit in meditation. The meditation practice should be done in the spirit of ease and comfort without force and suppression.

Om is the primordial sound to all mantras. The single syllable *om* symbolizes the supreme being. It pervades every space in the universe. Om is synonymous to the three sounds combined to make up *Aum*. The practice to coalesce the three sounds as one sound leads to Brahman consciousness. The symbolic sound *A* is the

Mind, Ayurveda & Yoga Psychology

creating force to all things, and *U* is the preserving force that takes place between the beginning and ending letter sound *A* and *M* respectively. The sound *M* is symbolic of the destructive force needed to transform what already exists into what is to exist in a new creation.

Aum is symbolic of the three personalities of the divine self—Brahman the creator, Vishnu the preserver, and Shiva the destroyer. These three representative forces play out the *Rasa Lila* or divine dance through the perpetual cycles of creation, preservation, and dissolution. The stage of the universe is the play of consciousness for the enjoyment of the supreme being.

The three syllable sounds of Aum represent the physical, astral, and causal plane respectively. Together, the sounds unite the three planes and bring one's awareness of the absolute self.

In the book *Mantra Shiromani*, Swami Jyotirmayananda relates the fourth aspect of Aum as *ardha-matra*, a half syllable that is represented by a bindu or point. It refers to the transcendental state wherein the three states of relative consciousness—waking, dream, and deep sleep—are transcended.

That state is referred to as the fourth only because you are counting the relative states of the other three. It is in itself pure consciousness. The consciousness of *turiya* never changes because it does not possess any attributes. The states of consciousness in waking, dream, and deep sleep continue to come and go in a cyclic manner. Wake and dream consciousness is associated with attributes, and deep sleep is the temporary loss of features; however, turiya is the permanent state of no qualities. Turiya can be associated to the unattached screen on which the three states of wake, dream, and deep sleep are mere projections.

Mantra

*Meditation changes how you
gather sensory information from
the outer physical world.*

The repetition of the sound of mantras has a definitive effect on one's consciousness. This can be attributed to the positive energetic vibrations being created within the person reciting them and to the surrounding atmosphere. At first, the sounds are restless and difficult to hold onto, but with repetition of the cited sounds and words, you will soften and become sensitive to the power of the mantra.

The sound of the mantra can be done in English or Sanskrit depending on one's proficiency in either. However, because Sanskrit is a pure phonetic language, the best effect would come from its natural form. It would be best to hear the correct pronunciation of the mantra sound by playing a recording of it or someone reciting the sound to you. Recordings can be easily purchase through the Internet and practiced in a particular space in your home. Over time the pronunciation of the mantra will become easy with better and longer focus on it.

Om Mantra

The repetition of OM can be done vocally and mentally with concentration on the center chakra point between the eyebrows, known as *ajna*. Om should be repeated with devotional feeling. Listen to it with attention in order to understand its intuitive meaning. It should be done with clear focus, intention, and reverence to the higher power within the heart. Om should be done daily and regularly to get the most benefit from the living manifestation of the mantra. The mantra renders the mind still and fills it with the sattvic attributes of joy, peace, serenity and happiness.

Soham has been called the universal mantra. Soham is the natural pulsating movement of the lungs during breathing. With attentiveness on the breath movement of soham, one can hear the respiratory flow sound of the mantra on inhale and exhale. The syllable *so* can be heard on the inhale sound of breath and likewise *ham* on exhale. Together, the vibratory sound of soham corresponds to the pulsating movement that breathes life to the universe. The pulsating syllable sound of so and ham helps to regulate the natural flow of breath.

Soham means "I am that." The mantra should not be merely repeated in sound, but rather one should reflect on its higher meaning. The listening to the vibratory sound of the mantra causes the breath to quiet one's feeling, thinking, attitude, and mind-set.

Other mantras synonymous with soham include *sohum*, *hamsa*, and *hum so*.

Dr. John Cosby

Japa Mantras

Every mantra is a blend of bija letters or seed sounds. The bija sound is a tool to bring about expansion of one's consciousness by employing the power of higher sound vibration. Bija mantras are concentrated consciousness in themselves that give a specific action by the aspirant. Bija mantras are often utilized for wealth, health, and/or adversity, but they are mostly used to worship deities. The highest is to meditate the Divine Being.

Swami Jyotirmayananda, the founder of the Yoga Research Foundation, explains the mystical meaning of the following bija mantra.

Om Namah Shivaaya Mantra

- *Om*—This is Brahman (the absolute self).
- *Namah*—This consists of the sound letters *na* and *mah*. Na is negation, and mah is ownership. Nothing is yours or mine. Therefore, you should live with an increasing sense of surrender to the supreme.
- *Shi*—This is the goddess Lakshmi. (You can develop spiritual wealth and virtuous qualities.)
- *Vaa*—This is the spiritual expansion of consciousness.
- *Ya*—This is divine communion within the heart (root letter of heart).

The mantra *Om Namah Shivaaya* starts the progression of spiritual movement toward the self. With recitation of Om, you invoke the supreme being. The continuous sound of namah prepares you to surrender the ego or the falsehood of the self. The repetition of the mantra naturally develops aspects of virtuous and divine qualities. There is increasing spiritual expansiveness to the communion of the heart with the supreme.

Maha Mrityunjaya Mantra

In his book *Mantra Shiromani*, Swami Jyotirmayananda explains the following the mantra. "Maha-Mrityunjaya Mantra" means "a mystical verse that is the great conqueror of death." *Maha* means great. *Mrityu* means death, and *jaya* means victory. This mantra is often called the "Great Conqueror" because when it is repeated with deep feeling and understanding, it bestows liberation, which is the ultimate conquest of death, the complete cessation of the cycles of repeated birth and death.

Maha-Mrityunjava Mantra

Om Tryambakam Yajaamahe
Sugandhim Pushti Vardhanam
Urvaarukamiva Bandhanaan
Mrityor Muksheeya Maa-Amritaat

Translation: "We adore the Supreme,
who is the possessor of the three eyes
and three energies, who is the enhancer
of fragrance and nourishment. May

> we be liberated from the meshes of
> death, as a fruit is liberated from
> the bondage of creeping vines, and
> may we be led to immortality."

Om is the mystical formula for invoking the supreme self. *Tryambakam* references the three-eyed deity. Lord Shiva is portrayed as having three eyes. Two eyes see and sustain all the practical realities of life. They symbolize the horizontal vision of the practical world of time and space. The third eye represents the vertical intuitive vision that intercepts the horizontal, transcending this illusory world. *Yajaamahe* means "We adore or worship [that deity]." This is a process by which an aspirant unites his or her soul with the divine self. *Yajaamahe* indicates surrender, self-effacement, divine communion, and divine absorption. *Sugandhim* means "spiritual fragrance." The unfolding Spirit in the lotus blossom of the heart emanates a celestial fragrance that manifests in the form of cheerfulness, serenity, purity, cosmic love, compassion, and other divine qualities. *Pushti Vardhanam* describes Lord Shiva as the increaser of spiritual nourishment. *Pushti* means nourished, and *Vardhanam* implies increaser. The divine self is the one who increases nourishment as well as fragrance (*sugandhim*). *Urvaarukamiya* refers to a vinelike plant that eventually bears fruit, such as the cucumber or pumpkin plant. The individual soul (jiva) is like a bud attached to the creeping vine of the world. That world is described as a creeper because its many branches or tendrils catch hold of everyone through karmic entanglements. The bud of the individual soul eventually blossoms in the rains of divine wisdom and the showers of divine grace. *Bandhanaan Mrityor Muksheeya* translates as "Liberate us from the bondage of death." Death is the symbol of darkness that hampers the ultimate unfolding of the spirit. Ignorance of one's true identity is the source of death. Life is a ceaseless battle against death. Spiritual life leads to victory (the attainment of immortality). *Maa-Amritaat* translates as "Lead me to immortality. May I no longer be separated from the immortal abode of the Self, Brahman."

Thus, this short but powerful Maha-Mrityunjaya mantra is an exquisite flower in the garden of the Vedas. It bestows upon its devotees the enjoyments of the world as well as liberation.

Hare Krishna Hare Rama Mantra

The reverential mantra is referred to as "Maha Mantra" (Great Mantra). Vaishnava devotees chant the mantra with loving devotion and sweetness to Lord Knishna. The mantra combines the names of Rama and Krishna, incarnations to Lord Vishnu. The chanting of this mantra vibrates a positively charged sound that is spiritually beneficial to the consciousness of the individual and the surrounding atmosphere. Initiated Krishna devotees chant sixteen rounds of Maha Mantra on their japa beads each day. The repetition of the sacred letters (japa) of the divine names (Krishna and Rama) elevates their consciousness toward God realization. The final objective of chanting the holy name is to return to Krishna consciousness or back to godhead.

The repetition of the mantra can be individually done on japa beads or in a group chanting atmosphere (*kirtana*). Kirtana is led by a vocalized call and response of devotee chanting in a temple and festival. The bhakti temples of Krishna are filled with an atmosphere of ecstasy and engaged devotion.

Hare Krishna Hare Rama

Hare Krishna Hare Krishna
Krishna Krishna Hare Hare
Hare Rama Hare Rama
Rama Rama Hare Hare

This concludes the chapter on some common mantras that are chanted in silence with mala beads and in kirtana (group setting). This by no means exhausts the endless number of mantras that are recited throughout the world.

Part 3: The Science of Ayurveda

Chapter 8: Tridosha: Prakriti and Vikriti

Introduction

In this chapter we will focus on the health and balance of the physical body and mind through the principles of prakriti and vikriti and the influence that the three doshas have on them. Ayurveda uses the quality and quantity of the doshas to determine the state of health and disease of the individual. Prakriti represents health and balance when the doshas are in equilibrium, vikriti corresponds to disequilibrium state of the doshas.

The natural state of the body and mind at the time of birth is prakriti. It is the DNA blueprint of the individual, which remains permanent. The prakriti is unique to every individual, which ayurveda uses to categorize the constitution types of the individual.

The three dosha body types that make up the structure and functions of the body are called the *vata*, *pitta*, and *kapha* types. Again, the balance state of the doshas is the equivalence to health. The deviation of the doshas from the natural order of prakriti is called vikriti or the disease state. During times of disease, one must constantly bring oneself back to one's natural state to sustain the state of well being. The daily influx of stress and environmental factors can cause disturbance to health (doshas) and the beginning illness and disease. The knowing of the qualitative and quantitative doshas of the birth state of prakriti constitution (through pulse reading), one can measure any difference or disturbance of the current dosha(s) to assess the state of vikruti constitution.

Ayurveda acknowledge that the comparison of the quality and quantity of the doshas between prakriti (birth) and vikriti (current) constitutions of the person is an important assessment to the promotion of perfect health. The equivalent composition between the two *kriti* leads to the integration of health. On the other hand, the widening gap between the individual's prakriti and vikriti constitutions is manifested by the disturbance of the doshas and ill health. Thus, vikriti is the increase and decrease of qualitative and quantitative changes that represent the current constitution in relationship to one's conceptive prakriti constitution.

In ayurveda, each disease is treated according to the deviated dosha that makeup the individual's constitution. The key to treating a particular disease is identifying the deviating dosha movement of vikriti from the birth constitution (prakriti). Knowing the qualitative and quantitative change of the dosha(s) between the conceptive constitution and the current constitution of the individual substantiates a pertinent curative course so that one can rebalance the disturbed dosha(s). The recognition of the degree difference of the offending doshas can validate specific recommendation to balance through dosha type diet, herbal medicine, and change to harmful lifestyle behavior in order to help return health to the tri-doshas. Most importantly, is the choice of compatible food qualities to dosha types in order to reestablish the body and mind. The incompatibility of food substances to one's basic dosha disposition can fall the individual from well-being and disintegrate the physical personality.

Good choices of foods that are easily digested, absorbed, and assimilated into proper microscopic nutrients leads to longevity and well-being. The opposite in the failure of the digestive system to properly assimilate viable foods can prone the body to illness. Also, the choices of poor diet can lead to residual cellular build up of toxins from the indigestible substances that remain the body. The buildup of lingering toxic waste, if left unchecked, leads to deteriorating health and the start of disease. This will be discussed later in the chapter on nutrition.

The ayurvedic conception of health and disease differs from the Western model of disease treatment in that the focus is on assisting the natural processes of the body to promote self-healing and ward off unwanted disease. Ayurveda focuses on treating the underlying cause of diseases rather than on the signs and symptoms of disease. Western medicine has made tremendous progress in treating traumatic injury with surgical intervention and containing contagious bacterial diseases to prevent them from spreading throughout society; however, its medical system has had less than spectacular results in treating chronic disease like heart disease, diabetes, obesity, gastric disorders, cancer, and serious mental disease.

Dr. John Cosby

Tridosha: The Biological Forces

The three biological forces of vata, pitta, and kapha together form the theory of tridosha. The principle of tridosha recognizes that these biological forces control all of the structures and functions within the body. It is connected to the samkhya philosophy in that the biological forces of vata, pitta and kapha take on the predominate form and energy of two of the five gross elements (space, air, fire, water, and earth). Vata takes on the gross elements of space and air. However, the remaining three elements help to shape the biological energy but in a lesser degree. The tridosha system of categorization guides treatment in order to balance these impaired intrinsic energies in the body. When there is no interference, the equilibrium of the doshas reciprocates into healthy function of the cell, tissue, organ and systems.

The three doshas do not work alone, but they are interconnected to one another. And all must be present in some degree to form the functional activities within the human body. They perform their functions as related to the characteristic qualities of the five gross elements (earth, water, fire, air, and space). For instance, vata dosha is primarily composed of air and space elements as mentioned earlier. Vata literally means "wind "because of its light and mobile qualities. It is governed by the principle of movement. The downward air movement is necessary to excrete waste from the body. Pitta dosha literally means "fire" because of its manifesting qualities of hot, sharp, and penetrating nature. It governs the principle of metabolism and transformation to the conversion of ingested substances to energetic nutrients at the cellular functional level. Gastric enzymes are required to break food into microscopic size to be absorbed into the body. Kapha dosha literally means "water and earth" which refers to the state of cohesion and attraction. Its prevalent qualities of water and earth are representative of heavy, slow, oily, sticky, and soft. It is governed by the principle of density and stability, which help to form the structure of the body (bones and organs). Lubrication is necessary to keep the eyes from drying out and enable the moisten elasticity of lungs to expand and constrict on breath movement.

The Dosha and Their Qualities		
Vata	Pitta	Kapha
Dry	Liquid	Oily
Light	Light	Heavy
Cold	Hot	Cool
Mobile	Fluid	Viscous
Rough	Smooth	Smooth
Subtle	Penetrate	Dull
Erratic	Flowing	Steady

The qualities of vata are the lightest of the doshas. It is reflected in the elementary attributes of space and air that runs through most of the body. The lungs have small spaces in bronchioles, which allow people to inhale and exhale the air. The pitta qualities of hot and penetration is meant to convert one substance into another form. The gastric agents in hormones and enzymes (penetrating) are necessary to convert food substances into micro particles for bodily functions. Kapha qualities are the heaviest of the doshas. They solidify and build the framework structure (i.e., skeletal) of the body. Besides the physical characteristics, the three dosha characteristics help shape the personality of the individual. The doshas give expressions to the corporeal personality as well as the characteristic qualities to the mental persona of the individual.

Although each dosha is specific to its function, there are numerous combinations of the doshas, with their permutation characteristics giving even more functions. Together, the tridosha and its permutations characterize all of the physical structural and functional activities in the human organism. They preside over everything on the physical plane whether the substance is inorganic and organic.

Ayurveda acknowledges the role played by the tridosha in determining the state of health and disease. A person's state of health is based on whether his or her present doshas are in balance with what they were at the time of his or her birth period. For example, if we determine an individual's prakriti constitution to be pitta dominant with vata and kapha doshas in less quantities, it becomes very important that the person eat a certain diet and lead a particular lifestyle to primarily preserve the balance of pitta in the individual. Moreover, in a disease state, more emphasis will be placed on restoring the pitta dosha. The characteristic qualities of intensity, sharpness, and penetration, if not taking care of properly, can lead to psycho-physiological disturbances. The ayurvedic approach to health instructs us to return pitta to its quantitative and qualitative states of prakriti. Once this is achieved, the final goal is to create an even balance of all three doshas to establish a strong immune system and strengthen organism.

Vata Dosha

Vata is not physical air but rather the subtle energy of air and space. Its attributes are dry, cold, light, subtle, transparent, irregular, rough, and mobile. It is often given the term *wind* so people visualize the movement of air. Too much wind against the eyeballs dries them out. Wind felt on a hot and sticky day bring relief.

Vata's characteristic of motion enable cells to communicate with one another. All sensory impulses are moved by vata. The entire nervous system network is under the impulsive movement of vata. The automatic nerve impulse to expand and contract the heart chambers requires motility to move the cardiac muscles. Otherwise the chambers of the heart would pump no blood and transport red blood cell to nourish the cells. Inhalation and exhalation of oxygen by the lungs and the diaphragm movement is caused by the "in and out" force of vata. These are all under the movement activity of vata. The activity of the gastrointestinal tract to secrete enzymes and hormones across its walls is required of vata. The excretory system eliminates feces, urine, sweat, semen, and menstrual discharge by the downward action of vata to expel waste. The birthing mother's cervix dilates, and she pushes the viable fetus downward with force to allow the newborn to come out and take its first breath. The blink of eyelids, hiccups, speech, snapping fingers, bending at joints, and locomotion all require movement.

The rise of thoughts, perceptions, and feelings are moved by the subtle element of air. Prana ensures that the neural network in a human collects, processes, and stores sensory data in the brain. In summary, all movement of bodily and mental functions are ruled by vata.

Physical Traits of Vata

People with dominant vata personalities are generally smaller in musculature and body frame structure compared to pitta and kapha types. They are the lightest of the three dosha types. Their build is slender (thin) with a flattened chest. Their complexion is usually pale. Their joints and veins are exposed because they are thinner with smaller musculature. Their height is generally either extremely short or tall. Vatas usually complain of coldness in their hands and feet, and they have dry and cracked skin. Their eyes are narrow, darting everywhere, and they have irregular noses that are smaller or crooked. The arterial pulse is rapid, and the feel of it is like a withering snake. They have irregular bowel movements with a tendency for constipation.

Psychological Traits of Vata

The psychological characteristics of the vata-dominant personality are determined by the nature of wind, which tends to change the direction of a person's thoughts. These people are easily distracted. They show quickness in thinking and bursts of new thoughts. They grasp ideas and information rapidly, but their keenness fades over time with less retention compared to the other doshas. Their reasoning ability is poor because of indecisiveness when they are excessively tired. They are extremely creative and imaginative in their thinking when they are balanced. Otherwise, they lose concentration when they are bored. They are always looking for new attractions and excitement. Their thought and speech can ramble on with the wind. They are very talkative but fall to exhaustion over time. Their talkative nature follows them into sleep, and as such, they are prone to insomnia.

Vata Disorders

Vata's excessive wind causes physical problems within these individuals, such as rough skin, dry and coarse hair, brittle nails, cracked feet, dry cough and hiccups, thirst (because they do not drink enough water), little appetite, hard and dry stools, fatigue, insomnia, intolerance to cold, muscle spasm, tingling, and achy pain. Ninety percent of neurological deficiencies are related to disrupted movement. They are prone to becoming anxious, irritable, impulsive, moody, impatient, poor decision, low self-esteem, confusion, fear, and worry, and they easily fall to stress. Extreme disturbances can manifest into delirium, depression, panic attacks, chronic insomnia, obsessive compulsive disorder, and suicidal tendencies.

The Function of Vata in the Body

Although vata permeates the entire body, it tends to manifests primarily in certain locations within the body. The main seats of vata are (1) the colon and surrounding areas (i.e., pelvic), (2) the nerves, and (3) digestive canal. The latter is illustrated as - food is chewed in the mouth and passed through the esophagus tract into the stomach area. The continued downward (air) movement of the ingested substance through the alimentary tract is attributed to the constriction and relaxation movement of the gastrointestinal muscles (peristalsis) to push it downward. The open space of the alimentary canal is necessary to move the particles of food through the digestive system. The viable nutrients are then absorbed (push) through the walls of the intestinal tract to nourish the cellular bodies. After digestion of the viable nutrients, the waste properties of the food substance are passed along to the colon for excretion. It takes approximately eighteen to twenty-four hours for food to

Mind, Ayurveda & Yoga Psychology

pass from the mouth through the digestive canal to the excretion of the waste from the colon. Delayed bowel movements of days and weeks can cause the residual intestinal waste to become dry, rough, stagnant, and toxic, which makes it harder to move through the colon. The residual buildup can narrow and obstruct the space of the colon canal, which then makes it vulnerable to chronic constipation. That, too, can have severe adverse effects, such as, colon cancer.

Chronic constipation causes an increase in the blockage of vata, whose natural flow is downward and outward. When the natural downward movement of vata is obstructed, it moves upward and spreads the residual toxic waste to other areas of the body. Toxins that remain in the gut for any lengthy time rapidly proliferate bad bacteria that then attack and destroy the good bacteria needed to properly break down the digesting food. If this situation persists, it can lead to severe bloating, flatulence, and distention of abdomen. That can also lead to stomach and lower back pain and chest pain. This condition can develop into diverticulitis and possibly into colon and rectum cancer. Other aggravated conditions include retrograde headache, physical fatigue, lethargy, poor concentration, sluggish memory, and sleepiness. If constipation worsens over a period of time, medical intervention is required to force a bowel movement.

In addition to the colon, the nervous system is the other major seat of vata. The nervous system is responsible for transmitting biochemical messages across the pre- and postsynaptic junction, the communication site between cells, and the neuron activities of the automatic and central nervous systems. Physical nerve damage in diabetic neuropathy can cause anxiety, insomnia, nervousness, and distress with physical spasms, tingling, and burning sensations. The more serious derangement of the neuromuscular structure is seen in Parkinson's disease, essential tremors, muscular dystrophy, myasthenia graves, cerebral palsy, and polymyositis.

Pitta Dosha

The Sanskrit word *pitta* is described literally as bright, brilliant, glow, radiant, and shine. The attributes of pitta comprise the qualities of hot, sharp, penetrating, liquid, and intensity. Pitta is generally a heating resource in nature. It regulates body temperature through the conversion of food into heat energy. It regulates appetite in thirst and hunger, gives luminosity to the complexion of the skin, and is responsible for the warmth and pigmentation of skin. It is the measured action of the digestive fire of *jatharagni* (pitta), which determines the strength of the gastrointestinal tract to break down the biochemical components in foods and turn them into energetic nutrients to nourish and build the cells in the body. Pitta transforms the amino acids into the four neurotransmitters of dopamine, acetylcholine, serotonin, and gaba, which control every function in the body. The subtle fire element of pitta (tejas) gives the necessary light in vision. The action of tejas allows the projection of the mind to shine its light rays on the object. The light of the object is then reflected to the back of the eye in the area called the retina. The retina is composed of layers of photosensitive cells in rods and cones (colors and shape) that transmit the visual signals of the image via the optic nerve to the brain, where the information is converted into a comprehensive vision.

Physical Traits of Pitta

Physical traits of the pitta person incluse a medium build that lies between the light vata and heavy kapha type. These people have good strength and muscle definition. Their eyes are sharp and bright and sensitive to light. Their skin is soft with good luster and coloring. The hair is lustrous and healthy. Their hair tends to gray and bald early in life, usually in their forties. They tend not to gain or lose weight, and they often exercise because of their competitive nature. Joints, tendons, ligaments, and muscles are toned and flexible. Their vitality is good, and they have lots of energy. They have a good and strong sexual drive. Their bodily temperature is hot, and they tend to perspire easier than the other dosha types.

Psychological Traits of Pitta

Psychological traits are characterized by bright and sharp minds. They exhibit very good intelligence, comprehension, and discriminatory prowess. They learn quickly with excellent memory, and they have good focus and concentration. They are highly disciplined. They finish assigned tasks, have good oratory skills, and show good leadership qualities. They tend to be joyful, cheerful, courageous, determined, frank, and hardworking. They work hard and play hard. Because of their competitive nature, they will overexert themselves physically. They will exercise in hot weather, which is not a good time for them. They will want to take on multiple tasks simultaneously, which can lead to headache and tension. They tend to be type-A personalities. Their fervent nature can develop into hypertension, especially later in life. Their desire for hot and spicy foods will cause hyperacidity, gastritis, skin rashes, blisters, burning stools, and diarrhea. With disproportionately high pitta, they are prone to fiery emotions like anger, irritation, hatred, lust, criticism, frustration, impatience, aggression, negativity, competitiveness, and arrogance.

The Function of Pitta in the Body

Pitta is found in all metabolic processes within the body. The five main areas of pitta include the small intestine (hormones and enzymes), blood (red blood cells), eyes (vision), skin (pigmentation), and brain (conversion of thoughts).

The brain's gray matter is under the influence of pitta sadhaka. It metabolizes relayed sensory information, feelings, thoughts, ideas, reason, and experiences. Sadhaka metabolizes the higher functions of the brain. It is responsible for perception, comprehension, discrimination, critical thinking, and the development of awareness to the self. Besides the brain, ayurveda recognizes that sadhaka is also located in the heart. Allegorically, the equilibrium sadhaka in the heart expresses in serenity, creativity, intuitive intellect and wisdom. The adage "Think with your heart, not with your head" is an understatement.

Pitta Disorders

Disorders in pitta constitution can manifest in fever, toxicity, inflammation, skin infection, hives, laryngitis, eczema, cellulites, strep throat, and bronchitis.

Kapha Dosha

Kapha is prevalent within the elements water and earth. It is the heaviest of the five elements and slowest of the doshas. The qualities are cold, heavy, slow, soft, viscous, solid, liquid, and moist. It is whitish and transparent in color. It is sweet and salty in taste. Kapha is firm, dense, hard, and solid. It is anabolic and is governed by the principle of cohesion. They are strong, grounded, and stable in body form. Amino acids and proteins are constituents of kapha, which are the basic building blocks to all structures. The water element gives it the viscous and moist qualities. It gives flexibility to the tissues and organs of the body. It lubricates the lung walls to enable it to expand and contract on inhalation and exhalation. Without the subtle water constituent, the lungs would not move easily, and they would crack. The good cholesterol lubricates and permeates the cell membrane wall, which is necessary for communication between cells, the transport of electrolytes in and out of the cells, and the influx of nutrients and oxygen and efflux of waste to and from the cells. The unctuous quality of kapha provides nourishment and insulation to the synovial joints for protection and less wear and tear to the area of the knee, shoulders, etc. The dense bone offers the physical body structure and locomotion. The knees, legs, and hips allow the individual to move about from one space to another.

These people tend to have good appetite when it comes to drink and food. The element of water is needed for the surface of the tongue so that one can taste. Without moistness, there is no taste experience of food.

Physical Traits of Kapha

One of the physical traits is a strong and well-developed build. These people's chests are broad, and their skin is soft, thick, and smooth. Muscle and bones are well formed. They have the tendency to gain weight, and it's difficult for them to exercise. They have big round eyes that are calm and attractive. Their hair is dark, wavy, oily, and luxurious. Their speech is clear and pleasant. Their bowel movements are soft and regular. Their sexual desire is slow to arouse, but they have good stamina upon awakening. They perspire

Mind, Ayurveda & Yoga Psychology

moderately because of the coolness of their skin texture. Sleep is deep, and they can sleep the longest of the dosha types. They can afford to exercise more and sleep less. Their gait is deliberate but graceful like a swan.

Psychological Traits of Kapha

Psychological traits show that these individuals are patient, loving, compassionate, tolerant, loyal, and giving to others. Their approach to life is mild and gentle. In balance, they are relaxed and easygoing in nature. Stability is important in their surroundings. They are slow to all changes. They are slow to frustrate and anger until they are pushed to the limit. Kapha types comprehend slowly, but once they have learned something, they retain the knowledge. Their memory base can be compared to an elephant who never forgets. They are comfortable with routine tasks. They make good managers because of their good communication skills with others.

In excess, the water element is retained and can cause edema, congested heart failure, mucus buildup in common colds, nasal congestion, productive cough, and asthma. They are prone to type-two diabetes, high cholesterol, and obesity. They are at risk of atherosclerosis, the hardening of the arteries. Lipoma and tumors are characteristic of kapha disturbance. Kapha imbalances can cause the rise of psychological characteristics such as greed, selfishness, possessiveness, and attachment. Their minds can become sluggish and heavy in thought, which make them at risk for lethargy and depression. They can become lazy and unenthusiastic in their outlook with others.

Kapha plays an important role in the stability and structure of the body. The mahabhutas—water and earth—are responsible for the body's solidity and concreteness. The main locations of kapha are the stomach, mouth, joints, heart/lungs, and brain.

The subtle kapha in tarpaka is located in the white matter of the brain and the cerebrospinal tract. It nourishes and lubricates the nerve myelin sheath, meninges of the brain, the spinal ganglion nerves, and the cerebrospinal fluid. It nourishes and strengthens sensory and motor receptors so that signals are smoothly transmitted without resistance along afferent and efferent nerve pathways respectively. Kapha moistens and lubricates the brain organ to maintain a suitable temperature and proper pressure levels. It provides nourishment, fluidity, and flexibility for the protection of the cerebrospinal column. Tarpaka kapha lubricates memory recordings of perceptions and helps with the quick retrieval of those experiences from the memory database. The neurotransmitter acetylcholine is the physical aspect to the lubricating function of tarpaka kapha. Acetylcholine is essential to the functioning mechanism of memory function. Studies have shown Alzheimer's to be decreased of white matter and plaque development of areas to the brain. The progression of senile plaques is attributed to the dryness (decrease acetylcholine), hardening and atrophy of the brain.

Prakriti Constitution Physical Characteristics		
Vata	**Pitta**	**Kapha**
Body Frame		
tall or short, thin	medium frame	robust and heavy
Skeletal		
bony, prominent joints	strong, symmetrical	thick bones and joints
Veins, Tendon		
prominent veins	moderate, flexible	hidden, thick skin
Weight		
thin to moderate, hard to gain	medium weight	heavy, subcutaneous fat, and gain easily
Body Temperature		
cold hand and feet	warm, hot, perspire easily	cool to warm
Skin		
dry, rough, cold	soft, oily, warm	soft, smooth, cool
Complexion		
pale, dull, plain	pink, copper red, flushed	white, pearl, oily

Dr. John Cosby

Hair		
dry, rough, coarse	soft, premature gray	thick, wavy, oily
Face		
small, thin	sharp, warrior like, angular	moon shape attractive
Eyes		
small, darting	medium, sharp, light color	big, white and round shape
Nose		
crooked, thin, beaked	medium and straight	thick, big, and wide
Neck		
thin, long or short	medium length	thick and bull-like
Teeth		
irregular, crooked, and small	medium and straight	big, strong, white, healthy enamel
Chest		
flat, protruding ribs	medium, define muscular chest	large, broad, barrel chest
Arms/Legs		
thin, long or short	defined, moderately tone muscular	thick, strong, solid

Hands/Feet		
thin, bony, crooked joints	medium and defined	large, firm, smooth

Nails		
brittle, cracked, rough	medium, pink color and strong	large, soft, thick and shiny

Appetite		
irregular, variable	strong and regular	steady

Thirst		
variable, forgetful at times	thirsty, drink excessively	tend to drink sugary beverages

Sweat		
slight perspiration	perspire profusely with smell	slightly sweat

Bowel Movements		
irregular, scanty, dry gaseous, prone to constipation	regular, soft stool, banana shape, yellow to light brown color, prone to diarrhea	soft, solid and prone to mucus buildup

Urine		
colorless, scanty, little	smooth flow, yellowish, warm sensation	steady and white color

Digestion		
irregular, light, variable	strong, metabolizes well	steady, strong, can be sluggish
Speech/Voice		
fast, talkative, chatter	sharp, authoritative, decisive in talk	soft, slow, gentle, and pleasant
Sexual Drive		
variable, quick, fantasy	intense, passionate, and controlling	steady, slow to start
Strength/Energy		
erratic, tire easily, stamina short term	excellent stamina, and competitive	steady and strong
Menstrual Cycle		
spotty and irregular	regular, heavy bleed, painful, PMS	smooth flow
Mental Orientation		
restless, passionate-oriented	Task-oriented	slow and sturdy at task
Memory		
quick learner but easily forgets	excellent retention of facts	long-term memory

Emotions		
fear, insecurity, and susceptible to nervousness	tend to be hot temper, can become aggressive	possessive of feelings, supportive and caring when balanced
Thoughts		
Changes, restless	sharp, penetrating and discriminate	steady and strong
Concentration		
short span, changeable	sharp and focused to detail	good and steady
Deep Sleep		
variable, light, disturbed sleep for less than six hours	good and sound sleep for six to eight hours	long, deep, and undisturbed sleep for eight hours or longer
Dreams		
flying, fear, plenty of activity	intense, vivid, lucid	deep sleep, and few dreams

This illustrates the physical, physiological, and psychological characteristics as related to the prevalent and variant combinations of the doshas. The disposition and outlook on life is variable among people. Given a small population, there are noticeable differences in feeling, perception, thought, and response among the individuals. No two persons are identical and similar. This explains why even two persons will react differently to foods, weather, relationships, stress, energy, stamina, and everyday situations. One person wants the heat turned up while another wants it turned down in the office space.

Knowing one's prakriti constitution offers the individual the opportunity to optimize his or her health. Prakruti can be thought of as the blueprint or genetics that makes up one's physical and psychological aspects. By knowing the dominant physical and psychological traits one can gain awareness to his or her self and surroundings as well as the proper food choices, sufficient exercise, sleep needs, adjustment to season changes, regular detoxification and rejuvenation regimens, and mindfulness practice for thought, concentration, and meditation, all of which can encourage a stronger, more flexible, and healthier personality. In conclusion, the implementation of a sattwa lifestyle can bring about balance, which translate into a harmonious personaility.

When one lives life according to his or her prakruti constitution, the person tends to live a joyful and contented existence. Prakruti is the conceptual state of mind and body. It is nature's innate physical and psychological disposition. Ayurveda's main goal in regards to health is to achieve a balance in prakruti constitution. The other important principle that pertains to health involving restoring the abnormal state of disease or vikruti back to equilibrium.

Vikruti

Ayurveda viewed health and disease as two phases of life. Life is the preservation and promotion of good health (prakriti) and the prevention of the disease state (vikriti). Svasthya (health) is equilibrium while vikara (disease) is chaos in the body and mind.

Vikruti is associated with the word vikara (disorder) or pathological manifestation. It is any physical, physiological, and psychological change from your prakruti or birth constitution.

Vikriti is the current distance away from your birth state. It can be viewed as the degree of difference from your conceptive constitution. The greater the degree changes, the more severe the disease state. The dance of vikriti mean you will encounter the inevitable distressors along the journey of time. The outside intangible factors (flu season) are given the chance to impose their muddle play on the mind, and if we neglect them by not fortifying our health, these can manifest changes and make us susceptible to illness and disease.

Vikriti disorders manifest in bodily disturbance in dhatus (tissue), digestion, excretion, ama (toxin), and the mental state of the individual. The primary cause that underlie the manifestation of vikriti disorders lies in the disturbance of the tridoshas.

Vata Vikriti

Any increase qualities in dry, rough, mobile, subtle, light, and irregular will bring on vatagenic disorders. The vata type is more prone to vatagenic disturbance than the pitta and kapha types. The higher the quantitative changes involved, the greater the severity of the vatagenic disorders.

Sign and symptoms of vata physical and physiological vikriti include difficulty in gaining weight, painful and stiff joints, chronic constipation, backaches, tremors and spasms, heart arrhythmia, dry and cracked skin, nerve disorders with paralysis and numbness, gastric paresis, shortness of breath, bronchospasms, anorexia, insomnia, somatic mood swings, excessive chatter, ADHD, fatigue, loss of energy, irritable bowel syndrome, poor circulation, and anemia.

Vata emotional and psychological vikriti can manifest as fear, fainting sensations, difficulty speaking, emotional discomfort, dry voice, lack of fluidity and creativity in thought, and desensitized to feelings. In mobile, you can see such characteristics as hyperactive, nervous, restless thoughts, excessive chatter, loose thought, and lack of focus. In rough, you can see such characteristics as worrisome, dry voice, insensitive feelings, impatience, indecisive expression in thoughts, difficulty in conversation, irritation, insecurity, and lack of concentration. In cold, you can see such characteristics as emotionally shut down, closed heart, unemotional and coldness in conversation, worry, and distance with self and others.

Pitta Vikriti

Because of pitta's fiery nature in intensity, burning, hot, sharp, penetrating, and liquidity, any quantitative change can intensify into pitta disorders.

Pitta physical and physiological vikriti include an increase or blocked pitta qualities, which can show up in loose and watery diarrhea, acid reflux, tonsillitis, inflammatory bowel syndrome, esophagitis, ulcers, UTI, acne, cellulitis, migraine headaches, conjunctivitis, retinitis, sinusitis, hypertension, PMS, septic joint inflammation, peptic ulcer, gastritis, high fever, inflammatory asthma, bronchitis, fainting, jaundice, skin very warm to touch, colitis, poison ivy and general skin rashes, neuritis, and otitis media ear infection.

Pitta emotional and psychological vikriti include the attribute of *hot* - hot headed, anger, frustration, emotionally blocked, argumentative, lack sensitivity, and shut down emotionally and hostility. Can become controller, difficulty letting emotion go in moments of intensity, visually want to complete all task at once, lack sensitivity to others, and intolerance. *Penetrating*—overly intellectualizes, heart is closed, words are stabbing and can be hurtful, sharp tongue, jealousy, opinionated, critical, egotistical, judgmental, and lack compassion. *Oily*—avoid emotions, detached, self pity, sharp thoughts, and thick skin.

Dr. John Cosby

Kapha Vikriti

This manifests in excessive qualities of sluggishness, slowness, heaviness, fluidity, denseness, and solidity. Because of its dense and slow nature, it tends to congest and obstruct when not in balance.

Kapha physical and physiological vikriti include the following: Kapha obstruction can appear in bowel obstruction, polyps, tumor, lipoma, edema, swelling of joints, congested heart failure, heart blockages, pulmonary edema, swollen ankles, glaucoma, weight gain, diabetes, obesity, polycystic ovaries, kidney stones, abscesses, mucus buildup, clammy skin, fungi infection, nasal congestion, fatty liver disease, hydroceles, and ganglion cyst, and mental symptoms can appear in lethargy, sluggishness, and sedentary lifestyles.

Kapha emotion and psychological vikriti characteristics: *Slow*—heavy and sluggish thoughts, bent up emotions, grief, dull, slow in response, slow to mentally absorb, and lethargy. *Dense*—stubborn, sadness, unforgiving, isolate emotions and thoughts, unwilling to change, stuck in thoughts, drowsy, depression, and emotionally heavy. *Cool*—emotionally shut down, detached, unloving, impatient, unsentimental thoughts, distance from others, and emotionally alone. *Soft*—shows in shallow heartedness, low self esteem, self pity, sluggish thoughts, unable to decide, sad, sorry for self, and seek others for strength. *Oily*—lethargic emotions, clingy, stuck in thought, blocked insight,

Mind, Ayurveda & Yoga Psychology

unclear in ideas and communication, slow in action, and sticky feelings.

Qualities of Vata, Pitta, and Kapha		
Vata	**Pitta**	**Kapka**
Light	Light	Heavy
Quick	Penetrating	Slow/Slimy
Rough	Smooth	Smooth
Clear	Sharp	Cloudy
Cold	Hot	Cool
Dry	Oily	Viscous
Soft	Liquidity	Hard
Mobile	Spread	Static
Subtle	Semi	Gross

The excessive intake of acidic, fermented, sour taste in foods can uprise into fiery emotions such as lust, arrogance, jealousy and anger. It feeds the needs of the emotions to stay and feel alive, and fuel satisfaction to the makeup of the mindset of the person, whether knowingly or not. The heating energetic effect wants to rise and expand in all possible directions. It wishes to fill space and forcefully spreads into other areas that allow it too. To illustrate, the increase of debris in acidity and toxic substances is force to overflow into the bloodstream where it is allowing to spread noxious waste to cause chemical changes to the structure of other parts of the body. The weaken area of the body now becomes compromised to futuristic disease.

Ayurveda emphasizes the use of the opposing guna qualities in the prevention and treatment of acute and chronic diseases. For instance, the treatment of heated skin with opposing cooling quality neutralizes the offending effect. Many ayurveda cooling herbs and applications to the skin have bitter and astringent properties, which means they constrict and cool. Cooling topical skin agents include aloe vera gel (considered the best), sandalwood, neem, rose, amalaki, and manjistha, among others. Manjistha is a powerful ayurveda herb taken internally to cleanse the impurities in the bloodstream. It can also be used in a poultice application with other herbs and rose water to treat skin disorders. The anti-inflammatory natural herbal licorice is recommended to relieve blisters and vesicle conditions (poison ivy) as well as recurring itchiness. Caution should be taken if licorice is orally consumed over long periods of time. One should monitor potassium levels because licorice can raise these level with prolong use. Ayurveda uses additional cooling herbs like guducci, brahmi, saffron, tulsi, and shatavari, which have anti-pittagenic properties and are used in the treatment of heated skin ailments. These are suggestions, and one should only pursue them under the guidance of a qualify physician and practitioner of them.

Chapter 9: Ayurveda: Digestion and Sapta Dhatus

Introduction

In this chapter, we will look at the nutritional science of ayurveda and the importance in diet to promote balance between the doshas. We will begin this chapter on the explanation of *ama*. Ama is described as the buildup of undigested foods that remain lodged in the body's tissues. This build of waste becomes toxic overtime and exposes the body to manifest disorder in the body. Initially, they manifest as acute episodes but in time progress to chronic stages of diseases. Next, we will discuss the seven bodily tissues (sapta dhatus) that make up the entire function and structure in the body. We will show the importance of a strong digestive system to efficiently breakdown ingested foods to viable microscopic nutrients to feed the bodily and mental constituents. It is the digestive production of the seven tissues or dhatus that produces the subltest matter in ojas. The life energetic sustenance energy of ojas is essential for the vitality and vivacity necessary to optimize the operation of the bodily constituents and subtle mind.

Ama

Low agni or digestive fire is a major cause of foods left undigested (ama) that remain in the body. The digestive fire is not strong enough to breakdown the ingested food particles into micro-nutrients substance for absorption and assimilation at the cellular level. In conjunction, the choice of wrong foods and disharmony in life style help facilitate the existence of ama. As ama is allowed to increase and deepen in the tissues, does it begin to overflow from its residence and spread to other weaken bodily areas.

The characteristics of ama substance are similar to kapha—cold, sticky, slimy, thick, slow, heavy, and unctuous. These impure qualities of ama are heavy and slow and when vitiated are easily stuck in weak spots of the body. When increased, these qualities tend to buildup and obstruct the channels of the body, such as the flow of prana along the nervous circuity. These toxic buildup compromise bodily functions and eventually lead to damage the integrity of the area lodged in, that can eventually manifest as chronic diseases. For example, the buildup of toxicity in bones can show in arthritic changes based on poor choices in eatery, low digestive fire, poor lifestyle, lodged metals, suppressed and unresolved emotions, which culminates in a weaken immune system that all have an affect on the integrity of the bone matrix. These are inappropriate behaviors that can lead to the detrimental effects of increased toxicity in *ama*. The buildup of ama can overflow the boundaries of tissue and organs, causing agitating physical and mental symptoms of dullness, sluggishness, laziness, dizziness, trouble concentrating and recalling, and poor reasoning and comprehension.

Mind, Ayurveda & Yoga Psychology

Symptoms of ama can show up in bloating, flatulence, abdominal tenderness, shortness of breath, headache, nausea, vomiting, constipation, myalgia, low backache, bad breath (halitosis), foul odor, and smelly stools.

Strong agni characteristics of hot, penetrating, sharp, and light oppose the thicker qualities of ama. Therefore, an important treatment in ayurveda is to eliminate the buildup of ama by the increase of the digestive fire in jatharagni. In conjunction to reigniting jatharagni, remedial therapy must start first with detoxification to purge the residual of ama, and then proceed to rejuvenate the body. Lifestyle changes, diet, fasting, herbal enema, oral herbal therapy, yoga, and meditation are effective measures one can take to get rid of ama.

Because ama characteristics are similar to kapha, herbal therapy uses the opposing qualities of bitter, astringent, and pungent to purge it. This bitter component helps to constrict ama into smaller substances lodged in the *srotas* (channels) in order to make expulsion more easily. The action of pungency is to strengthen the tissue agnis and to metabolize the offending toxicity by *cooking* the ama to dislodge for excretion. The healing action of astringency is similar to the effect of the bitter, compressing the buildup of the mucus membrane lining in order to reestablish integrity to the area.

And for this reason, ayurvedic diagnosis and treatment often begins with an assessment of the digestive process (jatharagni) that translates into a healthy constitution.

Dr. John Cosby

Sapta Dhatu—Seven Bodily Tissue

Health is the equilibrium of bodily doshas or biological humors. Healthy doshas are directly related to how food substances are properly digested, assimilated, and absorbed into bodily constituents. Ayurveda describes the potency in *jatharagni* as the strength of digestion to feed the doshas for health. Jathatagni is the gastrointestinal fire needed to completely breakdown large food particles into viable micronutrients to support the structures and functions of the body. The strength to the structure and function is directly related to the strong digestive power to nourish the sapta dhatus or seven tissues.

The Sanskrit word *dhatu* means "to enter into the formation of the body." Dhatu literally means "to nourish and support." Each of the seven dhatus is made up of infinitesimal cells (paramanus) that help to keep up the operations, functions, and structures of tissues.

The seven tissues are

1. rasa (chyle),
2. rakta (blood),
3. mamsa (muscle),
4. medha (fat),
5. asthi (bone),
6. majja (bone marrow), and
7. sukra/ arthava (male and female sexual fluids).

The series of sapta dhatus is regulated by its own digestive fire (i.e., rasa dhatvagni), which is

Mind, Ayurveda & Yoga Psychology

dependent on the overall strength of the digestive fire in jatharagni. The final product of the sapta dhatus collectively converts the substance into the subtlest physical nutrients called *ojas*. It is this refinement of ojas that nourishes the doshas and dhatus and keeps them balanced and optimize the processes of the constitients. We will explain latter to how ojas crosses over the physical plane at the heart area to nourish the subtlest matter in mind.

Ayurveda explains that when food is eaten and digested properly, it is transformed into these seven tissues that comprise the functional and structural makeup of the body. First, food must be transformed into chyle (micronutrients) before it can be transformed into rasa and then blood. And then from blood, it can produce muscles and other tissues.

Each of the seven dhatu has its own agni to process viable nourishment in order to feed itself and expel the waste products. After nourishing itself, the unused viable nutrients are passed onto the next dhatu agni in order to feed and transform into that tissue content. For instance, rasa dhatu passes along its unused viable nourishment to rakta dhatu, which further digests the substance and assimilates it into the constituents of blood tissue. So a portion of the previous dhatus' unused viable nourishment is converted into the current dhatu content and then the remaining unused viable nutrient is passed along to the next dhatu, and so forth. For example, the transformation of mamsa dhatu receives viable nourishment passed along by the previous two dhatus in rasa and rakta. The viable substance is further digested by mamsa dhatu agni to refine the nutrient contents so that the body can convert nutrient to build muscle tissue. Thus, the collective digestive process of the nutrient contents of the dhatus in rasa, rakta, mamsa, meda, asthi, and majja results into the final and seventh tissue makeup of the sexual fluids in sukra/arthava dhatu, which generates life form for the human race. The series of the seven dhatus must be properly digested by their own agni to transform into healthy sukra/arthava dhatu. The sequence of the seven dhatus cannot experience any impairment or breakage along the series of the dhatu. For example, if there is interruption in the process of asthi (bone) dhatu, then the following dhatus of majja and sukra as well as asthi dhatu can be impaired. Consequently, the interrupted transformation of bone tissue can manifest in deformities in bone structure (arthritis) or porous bones (decrease of calcium), osteoporosis or perhaps even compromise the integrity of bone marrow within the central canal of the bones. Bone marrow produces red and white blood and platlet cells. Any deficiency of mature red cells along with low white blood cells and decrease platelet cells can have a detrimental effect on the immune system (i.e, aplastic anemia). In addition to the impairment to ashti tissue, it may compromise the tissue development of muscles (majja) and reproductive cells (sukra/arthava) from being optimal.

Any impairment to the digestive process of the dhatus can be attributed to the buildup of toxins (ama), which may be caused by both low tissue digestive fire and lower jatharagni fire, the major digestive fire of the gastrointestinal site. The diminished fire of jatharagni reduces its ability to adequately heat cook, and breakdown the ingested food to feed the tissues. The reduced prowess of jatharagni and the much needed micro-nutrients will have a negative effect on the strength of the seven dhatu agnis to digerst and assimilate nourishment to the seven tissues.

Rasa Dhatu—Water Element

Rasa is chyle, plasma/serum, and lymph. Rasa is the essence or nector of food substances that is fed to rasa dhatu, which is then distributed to nourish all other tissues. Rasa is composed mostly of the watery element (jala or ap). Rasa is the major constituent of the body as it maps 60 to 70 percent water of the body. Its fluid portion shifts into all bodily space, including extracellular and intracellular compartments.

Healthy rasa gives feelings of happiness, joy, and contentment. It promotes a healthy mind. It gives brightness and lucidity to thought.

When present in excess, there is an increase in phlegm/mucous discharge, saliva, and edema, lymphadenopathy, low appetite, and fatigue. Chronic conditions can also arise, including congestive heart failure in association with defective mamsa dhatu function (workings of cardiac muscle), which may lead to myocardiac attack, pleural effusion, compromise to lung muscle, causing respiratory distress.

Reduced rasa can mean dryness, debility, dehydration, tiredness, rough skin, and fissure.

Rakta Dhatu—Fire Element

Rakta is blood tissue. It is predominance of tejas (subtle fire). It is the fluid tissue that circulates nutrients to the whole body. Rakta dhatu consists of cellular constituents that make up blood. It functions as one of the basic life-support systems of the physical body. Blood cells transport oxygen and nutrients to the infinitesimal cells of the body, and they also expel waste and toxic gases. It gives the skin and eyes their shine and color. It promotes good intelligence and discrimination. Healthy rakta promotes cheerfulness and exuberance. It passes through the heart to express joy and love.

One with excess rakta can develop disorders in heptomegaly and splenomegaly, hypertension, inflammatory abscesses, celulitis, burning sensations, gastric ulcers, hepatitis and jaundice. Decrease in blood constituents may develop into anemia, low blood pressure, fever, fatigue, infection, headache, and liver disorders. Blood that is deoxygenated can cause multiple illnesses, such as hypoxia, confusion, and delilium.

Mamsa Dhatu

Mamsa is muscle tissue. Earth is the predominant element. It is responsible for the muscular structure of the body. It protects the internal organs and the cardiac muscle, which regulates the pulsating heart. Muscles coordinate with bones to allow for the smooth movement of body parts. Mamsa gives strength, stability, stamina, and vitality to the body. Muscles are often associated with strength of mind, bravery, self-confidence, and valor.

Impairment in muscle tissue could mean tumors, fibroid, and mental aggression (from excessive steroid use in bodybuilders). Deficiencies may show an emaciation of muscle, fatigue, limb weakness, reduced coordination, the feeling of insecurity, and a lack of courage.

Medas Dhatu

Meda is adipose tissue, mostly fatty substances. Earth and water are the predominant elements. Its function is to give insulation and lubrication to the vital organs (brain, spinal cord, and nervous system). Adipose tissue stores potential energy. It insulates and generates body heat. Good cholesterol means fatty cells can repair and build cellular membrane to sustain communication between cells.

Too much meda rises in obesity, diabetes, and tumor (lipoma), high cholesterol, and greasy skin, fatty liver disease, and fatty abdominal visceral, and it can also give way to laziness and sedentary life style.

Reduced fatty tissue shows up in nervous fatigue, weakness of body, enlargement of liver, crackling joints, low self-esteem, and feelings of obsession and possessiveness. Meda dhatu is transformed into ashti dhatu by ashti dhatu agni.

Ashti Dhatu

Asthi is osseous (bone) tissue. It is predominantly the earth element, which involves dense bone structure. It supports the structure and stability to the boney components of the body—femur (largest bone), tibia, fibular, humerus, radial, ulna, shoulder, knee, ankle, hands and feet bones, among others. It generates locomotion, gait, posture, and balance by the moveable bone joints (pelvic, knee, ankle joints). Its solid structure encases the brain (skull) and spinal column. Ashti tissues bear the bulk weight of the body.

Bone deficiency is seen in alopecia, osteoporosis, joint stiffness, weakness of bones, lower back pain, general bone pain, loss of calcium, decrease appetite and digestion, brittle nails, and the decay and loss of teeth. There is a feeling of insecurity, a lack of strength, and miscoordination of body parts from deficiencies too. Too much bone density results in heaviness to limbs, difficulty with body movement, enlarge skulls, and bone spurs.

Majja Dhatu or Nervous System

Majja is specific to bone marrow tissue and nerve tissue. It is kapha predominate because of the earth and water elements. The kapha constituent of majja nourishes all parts of the nerve cell (sheath, axon, dendrites, etc.) to establish all-in-one communication between neurons, a healthy central nervous system (ganglion roots) along the spinal column, and smooth coordination throughout the brain. The nervous system is a prolongation function of the brain.

Majja dhatu fills up bone marrow, the spinal cord, and the brain. Bone marrow proliferates red blood cells, white blood cells, and platelets, which are extremely important to the immune system. The mind depends on the brain and nervous system to operate the functions of the physical body. The sensory stimuli are reliant on the electrical circuitry of nerves to transfer objective impression to the higher mind faculty.

Deficiency of bone marrow causes the immune system and health to deteriorate.

Sukra and Artava Dhatu

Sukra and artava are the male and female reproductive tissue respectively. Water predominate sukra and artava dhatu. It is the end product of all of the preceding dhatus. Sukra is white, viscous, and liquid. Sukra is the male sperm, and artava is the ovum of the female reproductive fluid and contents. Its function is to nourish sexual tissue in order to procreate human life. It affects the autoimmune system and thus health.

Sukra dhatu is digested by sukra dhatuagni that then transforms into ojas. Ojas is the complete succession of the seven dhatus pathway without any interruption along each dhatu nourishment and transformation process.

Diminished reproductive tissue causes low vitality, strength, and energy, impotence, weakened immunity, and low sexual drive. The making of too much reproductive sexual fluid can lead to an overactive sex drive; ovary, uterus, and prostate disorders; and feelings of aggression and agitation. Sexual fantasies can urge one to seek unrestrained sexual practices, leading to the overindulgence and possible contraction of sexual transmitted disease.

Ojas is considered the eighth dhatu. It is an updhatu (added dhatu) to the sapta dhatus. Ojas is the quintessence of the seven dhatus. The succession of the seven bodily tissues produces the end product, which produces the finest and subtlest matter capable of feeding the mind.

Although the tridoshas are the root cause of disease, its the dhatus that hold the physical expression of one's pathological state.

Ojas

Ayurveda considers the production of ojas to be paramount to the sustenance of the physical, mental, and spiritual planes. It is the vital life sustenance factored into the matrix of the bodily constituents. Its permeating energy source gives vigor and vitality to the body and mind. The subtle ojas material crosses over the physical plane to nurture the mind. Ojas allows better expressions in feeling, thought, memory, and intelligence.

The production of ojas through foods provides energy to build the body's natural defenses. Ojas is directly associated with the development of a strong autoimmune system, which can combat infection, and fend off stress. Ojas helps to prevent the initial action of disease by inhibiting its manifestation to take hold. In its highest form, ojas provides the nutrients to maintain the whole health of the individual personality.

Ojas quality is cooling, fluid, viscous, smooth, soft, and clear. It is sweet in taste and whitish/reddish/yellowish in color. It is similar to kapha properties but much subtler in purity, and it optimizes every biological and mental function of the indvdiual.

The internal luminosity of ojas flows into the physical appearance of the person with a bright and shiny face, glowing skin, clear complexion, bright eyes, strong and toned muscle, body strength, aura expansion, and enthusiastic speech. A person with high ojas is energetic, full of vigor and vitality, complacent, and content in daily life. Ojas fosters the psychological aspects of love, patience, happiness, joy, bliss, calmness, compassion to others, and radiant personality. It allows the mind to function with compelling memory and concentration, clarity of thought, creativity, sharp intelligence, mental prowess, and emotional and psychological stability.

Ojas-Building Foods

Diet has an intimate connection to the formation of mind. Mind is nourished from the subtlest of digested food, which feeds ojas. In turn. To have a strong digestive system, to have the highest quality of foods, it is imperative to eat organic foods. Then you can derive the end product of ojas from them. The sankrit terms *sattvic* and *ojas* are interchangeable with the word *organic* because of their positive effect on the body.

There are three types of diet according to ayurveda. They are classified as sattva, rajas, and tamas. Sattvic diet is the best among the three types of diet. Sattvic foods are natural, wholesome, and highly nutritious. Sattvic foods are broken down with little effort and easily assimilated into bodily tissues. Sattvic foods that are properly prepared do not allow for the accumulation of toxins. Sattvic foods are fresh, simple, and easy to digest. They are organic and produced with the sun. Sattvic foods are unprocessed and fresh in taste. Their wholesome content gives one the feeling of lightness, cheerfulness, clarity, serenity, and joy. They give greater energy than other diet types.

Sattvic foods include goat and organic cow milk, homemade yogurt, buttermilk, ghee, veggie juicing, basmati, jasmine and brown rice, tapioca, jaggery, sucanet, raw honey, whole grains, raw and unsalted nuts and seeds (almond, sesame, pumpkin, pine, coconut, walnut), figs, date, raisins, red grapes, apples, peaches, strawberries, blueberries, and pomegranates. These

Mind, Ayurveda & Yoga Psychology

foods also include olive, sesame, and flax seed oil. So too, you can add cucumbers, squashes, beets, yams, sweet potatoes, okra, chickpeas, yellow lentils, kidney beans, broccoli, watercress, bean sprouts, black gram, mung beans, dahl, fresh ginger, cardamom, cumin, fennel, and saffron. Foods related to sattwa, rajas, and tamas are given in a later chapter.

Rajasic foods are stimulants that tend to bring about an increase in mental activity. Regular eating of rajasic foods can rouse nerve and mental issues. Rajasic foods create motion and passion. They tend to be mutated and chemical-based. They are unhealthy foods that drain the mind, such as caffeinated beverages, sweetened drinks, and artificial sweets, all of which are stimulants. Rajasic foods include sour pickles, sweet chocolate, sour grapefruit juice, malt syrup, fructose, sweetened lemonade, salty peanuts, garlic, onion, red hot chili, salt, and excessive additives. Fast foods are rajasic.

Tamasic foods are static, heavy, and dull. It is the worse of the three types of food to digest and absorb. Tamasic foods make one lethargic and sluggish, and they cause the mind to become fatigued, cloudy, confused, drowsy, and stagnate. The microwave causes foods to lose energy and freshness. Enzymes and vitamins are removed during this process. Fried and oily foods lose freshness. Packaged and frozen foods are away from the sun too long. Tamasic foods include burgers, pizza, heavy cheeses, thick and creamy soups, heavy and thick meats, alcohol (spirits and hard drinks), and sweets.

Objectionable substances are canned, processed,

reheated, fermented, stale, and left over. These foods have a tendency to lower ojas and fail to provide good and healthy nourishment. Foods of qualitative deficiency can cause a change in skin color, looseness and tenderness in muscles and joints, inertness in limbs, heaviness within the body, an increase in body fat, painful bones, swelling, headaches, poor digestion, a loss of appetite, slow and irregular bowel movements, the buildup of toxins, contraction of the common cold, and degraded immunity to fend off illness.

Ojas deficiency affects the mind, causing mental exhaustion, sluggishness, dullness, a lower adaptation to stress, forgetfulness, poor decision making, drowsiness, stupor, distraction, and obscurity of senses to perceive fully. Contributory emotional factors include anxiety, grief, worry, fear, nervousness, delusion, confusion, sadness, misery, mood swings, selfishness, and explosive outburst.

Depletion of ojas can be caused by the wrong lifestyle activities, including smoking cigarettes, frequent alcohol consumption, excessive sex, a lack of sleep, improper meals at the wrong time, too much exercise, sense overstimulation, negative thinking, resentment, grudges, sedentary lifestyles, late nights, excessive television watching, poor association, and untruthfulness to the self and others. These all have a detrimental effect on ojas.

Ojas is pure biological consciousness that transforms into mental consciousness. There are two types of ojas depending on site. The ojas in the hridaya or heart region is referenced as *para ojas*, which consist of eight drops that nourishes the mind. Para ojas first forms nectar drops in the fetus during the growth of life, and it does so until the end in life. Therefore, it is essential that para ojas be constantly charged with sattvic foods and a conducive lifestyle to continuously produce nourishment.

The second type of ojas is called *apara ojas*, which distributes nourishment to all tissues and cells. Ojas sustains the biological life functions necessary to run the entire human machinery.

Ojas and longevity go hand in hand. Through wholesome foods, strong digestion, exercise and yoga, conscious breathing, deep meditation, soundless sleep, positive thoughts, and good association, can ojas contribute to longevity. Sushruta attributes longevity with balance of the three doshas, seven dhatus, ojas, strong agni, and proper excretion of ama or bodily waste.

Chapter 10: Ayurveda and Mental Health

Introduction

Yoga and ayurveda offer complementary approaches and techniques for achieving states of well-being. The primary principle is to cultivate the qualities of sattva guna in purity in feeling, thought, and reason. The increase of sattvic positive energies sublimates the spread of the negative energetic force of rajas on the mind to bring balance to the whole personality. The disproportiately high level of rajas and tama guna are responsible for mental agitation, frustration, and misery.

So in the beginning part of the chapter, we will look at the three gunas and related mental health, and in the latter part, I will provide an observerable analysis of the three gunas attributes associated with personality traits as well as some practical things one can do to increase sattva qualities in one's life.

Ayurveda, the Gunas, and Mental Health

According to ayurveda, the root cause of mental disorder is the volatility of the trigunas (sattva, rajas, and tamas). The primary principle of curative therapy is the eradication of the mental disorder by identifying the disorderly guna and its imposing negative force on the mind. By identifying the offending guna, the observerable anomality in one's personality can be assessed and treated.

Ayurveda recognizes all mental disorders are related to the negative energetic effect of rajas and tamas gunas, which causes the mind to deviate in distracted thought and action, as weel as, dullness and heaviness in percetion. The pivotal force of disturbance lies in rajas' increase mobility. That greatly irritates the mental process of both sattva and tamas. Sattva wants to lie in peace, joy, and clarity in thought. Tamas, the heaviest of the gunas, when balance lies in contentment, kindness, and compassion with loving expression of self and others. Sattva and tamas neither move by themselves, but they become mobile when raja acts on them. When the activity of rajas intensifies in higer levels does sattva and tamas energetic forces become distorted in thoughts and the expression of personality traits. Mathematically, one can reason the increase degree of negative disturbance onto the quiescence lake of sattva and tamas depth of mind to the rise of the energetic wave affect of rajas' over them.

The dominant activity of the rajas pushes sattva further away from its natural state of clear perception and easy flow in thought movement. Psychologically, the sattvic mind becomes agitated and unfocused. One's thoughts dissipate to wandering, and the mind loses its capacity to stay clear and sharp in reason and judgment. In addition to its negative effect on sattva, the expansive raja pushes its negative influence onto tamas guna as well. Raja causes the heavier and thick qualities of tamas to become more onfused and cloudy in the formation of thought patterns to make good reason and choices.

The slowness and denseness of tamas obstructs the lighter and transparency state of sattva, which impedes the latter's ability to sincerely express simplicity and straightfulness. The lack of expression of truthful thoughts and ideas may lead the sattvic person to become frantically righteous in speech, thus distorting openness in feelings and thought. Also, this disturbance from raja increases tamas thickness so that one becomes sluggish in the digestion and assimilation of sensory information, the retrieval of memory, and the production of thought, which overall affects the psychological aspects to one's personality.

The trigunas are constantly changing in qualitative contents because of internal stress and external relationships. The predominant guna among the three moves the mind in the direction of its influence, although the others play a minor role. The direction of mind is associated with the positive and negative influences of the interplay and transaction of the three gunas. However, the *fault* to all mental conflict is related to the divergent forces of raja and tamas. With the increase of positive qualities in noble thoughts, virtuous deeds, and sattva lifestyles does it generate response to the negative attributes of rajas and tamas that repudiate them to regain mental balance. Here, the science of yoga psychology and ayurveda principles offers a practical approach for the individual to restore the gunas to poise the mentation through the benefits of a sattvic lifestyle.

Manas Prakriti

The term *manas prakriti* is the unique mental characteristics of the person at the time of birth. It is comparable to the genetic blueprint of the individual's personality traits. Manas prakriti helps to define the general and specific personality traits of the individual by observing the interplay of the three gunas and their intrinsic energetic forces on the mind. The mental traits become more pronounce by means of the pervasive influence of the dominant guna as well as and the interaction of the other subservient gunas but in a less significant part. The disposition of the guna(s) and their numerous variant traits are the driving forces in the development of one's mental features and personality.

Furthermore, unique to ayurveda is the concept of *manas vikriti*, which is used to denote any deviation of the present state of personality characteristics in comparison to the original mental traits of manas prakriti (conception). It allows one to observe qualitative and quantitative changes between the manas prakriti and manas vikriti. By noting changes between prakriti and vikriti mansas, a measurement stick device of sought is helpful to gain insight into differences between the two manas constitution. This provides a systematic treatment plan to manage susceptible and identifiable mental disorders and diseases.

Consequently, ayurveda placed great significance on the qualitative and quantitative changes between prakriti and vikriti constitutions, which helped to advance its psychosomatic and therapeutic modalities in order to help the whole person through tailored made treatment plans.

Mental Characteristics of Personality

Ayurveda placed great importance on the promotion on mental health. The ancient ayurveda physicians were instrumental in the developmental concept of manas prakrti or the genetic mental traits as related to the expression of individual characteristics and behaviors. Manas prakriti outline the psychological disposition based on the observation of the many different types of personality characteristics. They used the most common and probable features, such as intelligence, comprehension, awareness, concentration, memory, discrimination, decision making, task orientation, attitude, motivation, mental energy, temperament, communication, behavioral expression of self to others, spiritual growth, among others. The categorized personality traits helped to explain the different behavior characteristics amongst many individuals.

Moreover, it recognized the fact that the attributes of all human personality traits were influenced by the interactive forces of the three gunas. The different personality traits correlated to the broad possible combinations of the three gunas. The mixtures of the

Mind, Ayurveda & Yoga Psychology

trigunas manifested into the many names and forms of the personality traits and subtraits. The variants in each core group give way to the numerous characteristics in personalities seen in the world. Think about the countless variations of the human fingerprint. Each person's fingerprint is different. The individual's mental fingerprint is unique to that person in relation to others throughout the whole world.

The following chart illustrates the mental traits of the personality and the trigunas:

Mental Trait	Sattva	Rajas	Tamas
Overall Behavior	insightful and truthful	ambitious, passion, and active	slow-moving procrastinator and possessive of matter and thought
Intelligence	brilliant, discriminate, and penetrating intelligence	quick learner, and intelligent	slow and deliberate intelligence
Communication	clear, direct, insightful, and honesty	controller, and driven with passion	slow, heavy, and monotone
Memory	strongly retentive	varies, and forgetful	slow to remember, dull and cloudy
Willpower	excellent and sharply focused	variable, and self-centered	sluggish and languish
Mental Energy	radiant and bright	driven with passion, and expend easily	repressed and suppressed

Dr. John Cosby

Secure	courage and valiant	fearful and insecure	repressive
Fear	calm, courageous	timid and doubtful	lonely
Worry	straightful in outlook	tendency to worry	heavy thought, hard to change
Stable	clear in decision	varies, dependent on desire and passion	selfish needs (food, drink), neglect appearance and direction
Stress	mentality is clear and accurate, and reacts properly to stress	becomes easily frustrated, and fearful of failure	sulk and distance self from stressful situation, shield ego
Understanding	excellent, discriminate, and insightful	variable, and self-interested	dull, and slow to comprehend
Organized	strongly detailed	fluctuates, can be disorganized, too many things on the plate	selfish interest and hoarding which limits them
Judgmental	compassionate	envious	dark side
Irritable	clear and steady	frustration of material wants not obtained, and prone to nervousness	self-induced, which lead to heaviness and depressed moods

Selfish	generous, and gives selfless to others	selfish in wants and needs at expense of other	self-absorbed, and non-striving
Task oriented	clear and purposeful	tyrannical	gluttonous
Mental attachment	for the highest cause	passionate, and unruly cravings	greed and possession
Initiative	strongly, and highly motivated	burst of energy with each new task but tires	cloudy, slow, and procrastinator
Lethargic	bright and clear	variable, depends on interest and energy	prone to lethargy
Decision	clear, sharp and discriminate	quick decision making	indulgent behavior
Awareness	insightful	material	limited with self-centeredness
Intimate	loving and honest	self-absorbed	possessive and clinging
Focused	penetrating, sharp, and centered awareness	prone to distraction	cloudy and dull
Expressive	precise and straightforward	changeable to interest at hand	hold back, repressive
Depression	tend not to be down	tendency from frustration	tendency to moods

Love	clear and honest	personal gains and self-indulging	attached, clingy, and greedy
Discipline	self-disciplined	self-interested	gluttonous driven
Resentful	pure in thought	cruel/envious	dark side
Arrogance	purity and virtuous	consumed by self-interest	infatuated to possessiveness, gluttony
Spiritual Growth	compassionate and dedicated to righteous dharma	consumed with self-desire and passion	inauspicious and gluttonous

Review the previous mental trait chart to see where you lie in the mix of it all. Traits can cross over into another guna type/ column. Altough both sattva and raja qualities may appear to overlap, try to pick one that would be the more prevalent for you and the other guna secondary to the characteristic of the mental trait. At the end, tabulate the vertical column of characteristics to see which guna is predominant in you and which is not in describing your guna type personality.

The psychological traits can be described in terms of sattva, rajas, and tamas, which makes it easy to identify what kind of thoughts we show preference, the type of characteristics of the people we draw into our lives, and the play of circumstances around us. The goal is to balance the gunas with the intent to raise the predominance of sattva among the three gunas, which has a positive spiritual influence to sublimate the negative influence of rajas and tamas.

The predominance of sattva moves into the unconscious mind in order to keep the negativity of rajas and tamas from sprouting growth into the conscious mind. When sattva charactistics moves spontaneously into the unconscious mind, does positivity reflect into our waking conscious world.

Chapter 11: Diet for Vatta, Pitta, and Kapha

Introduction

In this chapter we will look at how different foods can be used to promote balance of health. In ayurveda, the way a food property is identified is by its taste (rasa). The defining of each taste is done by using the elementary properties of foods and their effect on the constituents of the body. Different tastes promote balance for different dosha constitutions. The understanding of one's natural constitution (prakriti), deviation from one's natural constitution (vikriti), and an understanding of the effect of the six tastes allows one to choose foods that promote balance of dosha types. Ayurveda classifies food in six different categories of taste and assigns various properties to each taste. So in this chapter we will be discussing these six different tastes, the particular taste found in the physical elements (*panchamahabhuta*) of foods, and the effects that each taste has on a person's constitution.

> "Plant give leaves, flowers, fruits, and stem to others. They do not enjoy any of these things for themselves. They lead a life of an ideal donor unconditionally."

Ayurveda through Taste

Ayurveda places great emphasis on rasa or taste in regards to the art of eating. Over the centuries the ayurvedic concept of taste and food has been integrated into Indian cuisine. The art of Indian cuisine has always made for tasty, pleasurable, and palatable dishes. The knowledge of taste and food types has been passed down for many generations of the Indian home. Homes used food, taste, and their properties to help nourish, build, and strengthen the family members. At times of sickness, the family instinctively knew what taste, food, herbs, and spices to prepare in order to eliminate the suspected illnesses and diseases.

> The body is the product of food, and disease arises on account of faulty foods.
> —Caraka

Rasa—Taste

The Sanskrit word *rasa* is closely translated as the word *taste* in the English language. The Sanskrit language is very expressive in communication. Thus, the connotation of the word rasa has multiple meanings, including nectar, essence, juice, ambrosia, bright, and others. The Webtser dictionary describes the word taste as "the sense of qualities and flavor of an eatable and soluble substance has directive of taste buds." Scientifically, the taste buds on the tongue give an impression that is sent to the brain to identify the substance for digestion. The ayurvedic concept of taste goes beyond the sensation instead to the recognition of the energetic action of food properties.

Western cuisine alludes to four tastes—sweet, sour, salty, and bitter. Ayurveda differs in the number of total tastes. It has six (adding pungent and astringent), and each helps to extend the concept to the energetic properties of food.

The six tastes are

1. madhura (sweet),
2. amla (sour),
3. lavana (salty),
4. katu (pungent),
5. tikta (bitter), and
6. kashaya (astringent).

The six rasas are shaped according to the quality and quantity of the mahabhutas constituents found in the edible substance. The predominance of the two elements of the panchabhutas in the food substance determines its unique taste and energetic action. Thus, the specific taste is related to the particular configuration of the elements, which lies dormant within the food substance until it becomes active when it touches the tongue. The food substance needs to touch the tongue for the food's *panchabhutas* to come alive for the perception of taste. The action of taste is forwarded to the mind so that one can identify the food substance, which then starts the process of digestion. It is the mind that actually perceives food while taste is the intermediate instrument used to connect the body to the outer food chain.

The theory of panchabhuta outlines a bioenergetic foundation for every food type and taste. It is taste that initiates digestion, absorption, and assimilation of food into the body, and this has a direct effect on the dosha(s). Thus, the right mixture of the elements in the foods could be applied to balance the doshas.

Ayurveda categorizes foods and their tastes along with their energetic effect on the dosha. For example, honey is mostly composed of the elements of earth and water, which gives the taste of sweetness (madhu). Its elementary attributes are heavy, unctuous, smooth, and thick. Its aspects are similar to kapha dosha. Thus, it has the tendency to increase the latter dosha type. The excessive usage and amount of honey therefore can increase the disturbed kapha dosha and make the body vulnerable to gaining weight, increasing glucose levels, and causing interference with glucose resistance and cellular function. Too much sweet (over time) can possibly cause diabetes and other kapha-type diseases. On the other hand, the right amount of honey and its therapeutic action of sweet taste can decrease vata dosha disturbances. This is because the sweet taste is grounding, smooth, unctuous, heating, stabilizing, and anabolic to the expansive, light, dry, irregular, rough, and cool innate qualities of vata.

Every taste and its energetic action will either increase or decrease the doshas. The dual action of

Dr. John Cosby

increase and decrease is similar to the acceptance of the universal law "Like attracts like." For instance, the taste of Greek yogurt is related to the quality of earth and fire, which give the distinct sensation of sour (amla). Its ingredients give excellent digestive enzymes and probiotic effects to help digestion. The fruitless and unsweetened yogurt is the best of the yogurts. But like anything, eating beyond moderation can create an unwanted effect. For example, too much sour taste will increase pitta and kapha doshas. The benefit of the sour taste will help decrease vata dosha by increasing the digestive fire, which may increase appetite and the want to eat more and gain weight. In summary, each taste is distinct to the configuration of the predominance element of a substance.

Light quality foods in rice cakes, cabbage, dry raisins, cottage cheese, and tofu will increase vata. The taste of dry and light resemble vata, and therefore, they have a tendency to increase vata. Hot, spicy, acidity, and fermented foods and beverage have the tendency to increase pitta dosha. To decrease the heating quality of pitta, cool foods should be sought to limit and oppose the expanding, heating, and sharp tendencies of pitta dosha. The consumption of buttermilk, unsalted butter, sweet apples, Medrol dates and unripe bananas are good food choices. Kapha qualities resemble heavy, unctuous, thick, slow, and cooling attributes and are thus aggravated by thick and aged cheeses, thick molasses, sweet cakes, ice cream, large portions of

Mind, Ayurveda & Yoga Psychology

pasta and garlic bread, high fructose content sodas, fried foods, and etc.

The six tastes, five elements, and their effects on the three doshas are shown in the following table:

Taste	Elements	Taste Effect on the Doshas		
		Vata	*Pitta*	*Kapha*
Madhu (sweet) rasa	Water and Earth	Decrease	Decrease	Increase
Amla (sour) rasa	Earth and Fire	Decrease	Increase	Increase
Lavana (salty) rasa	Water and Fire	Decrease	Increase	Increase
Katu (pungent) rasa	Air and Fire	Increase	Increase	Decrease
Tikta (bitter) rasa	Air and Space	Increase	Decrease	Decrease
Kashaya (astringent) rasa	Air and Earth	Increase	Decrease	Decrease

The sweet, sour, and salty tastes are the heaviest elements, and they help reduce the light nature of vata, while the tastes of pungent, bitter, and astringent are the lightest elements (vatagenic) and thus increase it. Kapha is just the opposite in action. The tastes of sweet, sour, and salty are kaphagenic, which aggravate kapha, and the three tastes of pungent, bitter, and astringent reduce and pacify it. Pitta is aggravated by the increased tastes of sour, salty, and pungency, and it is reduced by the tastes of sweet, bitter, and astringent.

It is the composition of the elements in a substance that gives taste its experience. The taste of a substance is generated by the composition of the prevalent mahabhuta and the combining lesser elements, which gives it a specific energetic effect. Cow's milk is sweet in taste and composed chiefly of the elements earth and water, although the remaining three of five elements exist in smaller and varying degrees. The energetic effect in sweet is *cooling*. Sweet acts on the body as an anabolic, tonic, and nutritious value to all seven tissues (dhatus). The sour taste of lemon is the primary elements of fire and earth. Its energetic effect is *heating*, and its action is to stimulate taste and increase digestive power. Salty taste (such as kelp) is dominated by the elements of fire and water. Its energetic effect is *heating*. Its action causes an increase in saliva, adds to taste, and aids in digestion. Black pepper is pungent in taste. Its energetic effect is *heating*. Pungency action stimulates digestion, clears the sinuses of mucus, cleanses circulation, and causes diaphoresis. Bitter taste is prevalent of the elements air and space, which makes its energetic effort *cooling*. Its action constricts and cleanses, and it is generally antibacterial in nature. Pharmaceutical dermatological products essentially include zinc oxide ingredients that are used topically to treat skin disorders because of its bitter action (constrict). The fresh gel of aloe vera is perhaps the best application for skin disorders. Astringent tastes are made up of the elements of air

Mind, Ayurveda & Yoga Psychology

and earth. The astringent substances in pomegranate and witch hazel are energetically *cooling*. The action of astringency helps to absorb and dry moist areas of the body (in the case of skin wounds). It is useful to stop diarrhea. Witch hazel used both topically and orally together can help to soothe and pacify mild to moderate varicose veins in the lower extremities when caught early.

The Six Taste Properties and Actions on the Physiological and Psychological States of Mind

Ayurveda saw the *energetic effect from food properties* as having a real influence on the function and structure of body and mind. The energetic effect of the exogenous substance could be applied to balance and restore the individual dosha(s) constitution. The panchabutas properties of a particular taste could be sought in food properties to increase and decrease dosha quality and quantity. On the other hand, faulty taste and wrong food choices give way to an increase in the disturbance of dosha(s). Thus, there is a direct relationship between taste, food substance, energetic properties, and their effect on the tridoshas.

Madhura Rasa

Sweet taste pacifies vata and pitta and aggravates kapha in excess. The qualities of heavy, unctuous, cool, and firm are similar to kapha and thus increase kapha dosha in excess. The attributes of sweetness reduce vata and pitta dosha. The elements of sweet taste are mainly earth and water, although all five elements exist in each food substance in varying amounts. These two elements found in sweeter foods are the heaviest of the five. It promotes the satisfaction of all seven tissues (lymph fluid, blood, muscle, adipose tissue, bone, bone marrow, nerves, and reproductive organs) or dhatus. It nourishes all the constituents of the body. It strengthens, stabilizes, and grounds the body and mind. It is pleasing and gratifying to the state of mind. It is a practical source of life energy (glucose) used to feed the brain and other major organs. The anabolic effect is most important during the growing years of childhood to adulthood. Caraka mentions that it is good for complexion, burning sensations, and hunger.

Of the six tastes, sweet is most similar in characteristics to ojas. The dairy product of organic goat, cow, and buffalo milk and ghee innately increase the subtlest matter of ojas. Ojas is the essence and nectar needed to promote the life source, energy, strength, and immunity of the body. Sweet-tasting substances include uncomplexed sugar, honey, raw cane sugar (jaggery), sugarcane, basmati and jasmine rice, ripe yellow banana, fresh juicy raisins, season coconut, wheat, potato, and natural licorice. The moderation of kapha quality food substance can be ingested to promote ojas. A warm cup of hot organic milk with five cardamom seeds and uncontaminated honey is a wonderful recipe.

The stagnation of heavy kapha foods (excessive) tend to impede the bodily channels (srotas) that prevent the free flow of ojas and prana. The low flow of ojas and the life forces of prana weakens the immune system (cancer, HIV).

When you consume a good deal of sweet chocolate, you become satisfied and full. The sweet taste brings satiety and delight, and it brings joy and happiness to the mind. Sweet is the most-sought-after taste for all creatures—insects, bees, monkeys, animals, and humans. Because of its calm and grounding effect, sweetness is sought by people in moments of agitation, nervousness, discomfort, insecurity, and hunger. One may have an adverse tendency to excessively indulge in the taste. In today's high-tech world, its negative by-product has brought on two of the fastest rising global epidemics—diabetes and obesity.

In excess, it disturbs kapha dosha which increases the risk to arise when we consider the possible manifestation of diabetes, renal insufficiency, obesity, liver fatty tissue, gallstones, coronary artery diseases (plaques), hyperlipidemia, high ama, candiadis, gastropariesis, worms, and lipoma. Sweet ingredients in lower value can be found in white flour, corn fructose (soft drinks), flavored ice cream, cakes, table sugar, processed foods, among others.

Mental symptoms appear as fatigue, general weakness, sluggishness, heaviness, laziness, dullness, and a lack of motivation.

Dr. John Cosby

Amla Rasa

Sour taste pacifies vata and pitta and aggravates kapha in excess. The taste is derived primarily from the elements of fire and earth. Sour is hot, unctuous, liquid, and heavy in qualities. Pitta dosha is aggravated by the hot nature of sour. Kapha dosha is disturbed by the water element retention mechanized in excess of sour. It pacifies vata dosha with its grounding and anabolic action. It increases digestive enzymes, which helps the vata person. It stimulates the senses and mind. Sour stimulates saliva and appetite. The taste in the mouth makes the tongue pucker and increases salivation for swallowing. It gives added satisfaction to food. Sour moistens, which helps break down substances easily into smaller particles that can then enter the throat and move downward. It adds taste to food and heightens the gustatory sense response by the operating brain. It ignites the digestive enzymes and hormones to begin digesting the food contents. The sour attribute of viscous moistens the walls of the colon, which helps in defecation. It strengthens the body and promotes health in mild to moderate consumption. Sour substances include miso, pickles, yogurt, buttermilk, fresh cheese (curd or paneer), unripe mango, fermented wine, lemon, grapefruit, and tamarind.

Too much sour may increase heating impurities in the bloodstream (rakta) and manifest in the eruption of skin rashes and hives. Because the blood directly feeds the skin, the excessive heating aspect of sour may exacerbate pre-existing conditions of psoriasis, eczema, urticaria, ulceration, and pustule to the epidermis and deeper subdermal layers. Overwhelming amounts of sour disrupt the normal integrity of the gastrointestinal mucus layers, which can also alter the flow of gastric secretions needed to break food down. Too much sour causes high acidity in the stomach and intestines, which can result in hyperacidity, indigestion, gastritis, ulcers, diarrhea, and intestinal inflammatory disorders (ulcerative colitis). Furthermore, because of its heating property, it can cause thirst, burning sensations to the throat and chest, itchiness, tingling, obstruction of the channels, toxicity in pregnancy, and a rise in blood pressure.

Mental disturbances manifest as headaches, dizziness, stagnation, sluggishness, dissatisfaction, envy, jealousy, and irritation.

Lavana Rasa

Salty taste pacifies both vata and pitta and aggravates kapha in excess. The qualities of hot, unctuous, liquid, and sharp tend to aggravate pitta and kapha doshas. Like sour, it pacifies vata dosha. It is primarily composed of the elements fire and water. Salt attributes are heating, heavy, and fluidic. It stimulates hunger, saliva, appetite, and jatharagni (main digestive fire in the stomach) to break down food into minute particles so they can be easily absorbed and assimilated. It reduces mucus buildup as a benefit. It removes blockages to bodily channels. Its moistening property acts as a laxative, which moves the contents along the excretory pathway. In mild to moderate consumption, it regulates kidney and urination function.

Next to sweet, salt is the second most-sought-after taste. Salt is widely used to preserve food. It is added in about every can of food and served in most restaurant dishes. Its long-term usage causes an addiction in the mind. Too much salt can camouflage the other five tastes. Throughout every culture we find salt in the form of table salt (NaCl), kelp, Irish moss, black salt, sea salt, seaweed, and rock salt. There are several rock salt types, but the black one is the most recommended because of its homogenous interaction with foods. Himalayan pink salt is considered the best as the body assimilates it well and it has a lower water-retention effect than other salts.

In excess, it causes retention of water, which obstructs the lymph nodes and capillaries. This consequence shows up as edema. It overloads the renal angiotensin/aldosterone normal mechanism, which results in higher retention of salt and reveals itself in congestive heart failure, kidney failure, high blood pressure, pulmonary edema, and renal hypertension (second leading cause to uncontrolled hypertension). It causes burning sensation and itchiness to skin, dries skin, overactivates the sense of taste, destroys the protective barrier of the stomach's mucus membrane, decreases semen and ovum reproductive fluids, and contributes to baldness and wrinkles.

Overuse of salt consumption affects the mind so that one becomes irritated, selfish, angry, jealous, fiery, self-centered, hateful, and unsatisfied. Salt is very addictive, so one easily falls victim to cravings.

Katu Rasa

Pungent taste pacifies kapha and pitta and aggravates vata in excess. It qualities are hot, sharp, light, and dry. It is primarily composed of air and fire. It increases vata and pitta doshas and decreases kapha dosha. It cleanses the mouth, stimulates the senses, especially taste, enhances appetite, increases jatharagni (enzymes and hormones) to aid in digestion, and reduces excessive buildup of phlegm, mucus, and edema. It can be used to reduce fat and weight loss, and it is good in eliminating high kapha. It aggravates pitta and vata because of its heating and dry properties. It kills worms and helps to clear mucus secretion in the throat and nose regions. Its energy is opposite to the taste of sweet in that it is heating, drying, light, and expanding in nature. Pungency is helpful in drying sinusitis and upper respiratory disorders. An old ayurveda formula is adding equal amounts (1/3) of dry ginger, black pepper, and Indian pepper or piper longum to a level teaspoon of pure honey spread on top to soften the swallow of it. Honey acts as a catalyst that helps to smooth the thick mucus of the throat and lung passageways. It also helps assimilate the former ingreients across the membrane of the lungs. Pungent substances include black pepper, chili peppers, pippili, horseradish, cloves, black mustard seeds, garlic, raw onions, radish, cayenne, asafaoetida (hing), wet and dry ginger. Of interest is the cayenne substance with attribute of heating, has an inherent property that cannot be clarified by science. It can be used in small amounts to pacify peptic ulcers. One would think that its heating action would worsen the inflammatory condition. Somehow it doesn't, and cannot be explained.

In excess, the pungent qualities of heat, dry, and light can weaken the natural barriers lining the body system. Spicy and hot foods can disturb the lining of the esophagus and its lower sphincter muscle where food leaves the esophagus and enters into the stomach. Misuse of spicy and hot ingredients can lead to acid reflux, medically diagnosed as gastrointestinal reflux disorder. Too many irritating and spicy foods can cause gastric ulcers, especially consumed at late dinners when the body produces less enzymes and hormones to aid in digestion. Constant and overwhelmed pungent foods will irritate and emaciate the stomach and small intestinal mucus membrane wall, which also destroys the good bacteria needed for defense and digestion. It can turn into diverticulitis, ulcerative colitis, hemorrhoids, and gastritis. Heat overflows into the bloodstream, which circulates out to the skin layers, causing burning and toxic rashes. Entry into blood vessels can cause the buildup of impurities, and those are then circulated throughout the body. Long-term use dries synovial fluid of joints and desiccates bony structure of fluids, which diminishes their density and structure. In excess it can diminish bodily fluids and energies.

Mental disturbances are exhibited by nausea, giddiness, gasping for breath, weariness, fatigue, fainting, dizziness, mental weakness, loss of consciousness, headache, dullness, heating sensations, and altered mental states. People who consume too much spicy food can be hotheaded and sharp with their tongues, as it feeds their emotional makeup.

Tikta Rasa

Bitter taste pacifies pitta and kapha and aggravates vata in excess. The predominant elements are ether and air. These are the lightest of the five elements. The qualities of light, dry, and cool are similar to vata dosha. Thus, vata is easily aggravated when used too much. The bitter qualities of constriction and coolness oppose the heating and expanding pitta dosha. The dry and light bitter qualities pacify the heavy and unctuous attributes of kapha dosha. It is used in skin disorders to treat rashes, poison ivy, hives, psoriasis, eczema, skin burns, and infections. In Western pharmaceutical preparations, bitter applications are used to reduce inflammatory skin diseases. Aloe vera, neem oil, goldenseal, bitter melon, manjistha, turmeric, and sandalwood herbal ingredient are used separately or combined in many ayurvedic skin preparations. Fresh aloe vera (not the lotions or moisturizes) is consistently successful in the treatment of many skin disorders (especially sunburn and irritating skin). Besides skin rashes, the bitter quality is useful in alleviating itchiness and dryness.

This particular taste action works to dry and narrow mucus buildup seen in congested allergies, sinusitis, and other upper respiratory ailments. It is used to treat fever, vomiting, and nausea. It promotes digestion by clearing the mucus membrane. Its characteristics are used in an ayurveda tonic to treat diabetes. For example, one can extract the juice of a fresh bitter melon and ingest one half to a full eight ounces in the morning. One should drink this tonic very fast, or the person should add something (apple juice) to it because the taste is very bitter. It detoxifies, strengthens, and rejuvenates the liver, pancreas (endogenous insulin), and circulatory system, which can help treat diabetes. The juicing process should be done for nine to twelve months for the best results. Moreover, bitter rids the body of parasites and worms, and it is a powerful antiseptic in nature. It is helpful in reducing edema and water retention. The bitter attributes of light and dry constrict and oppose heavy and moist conditions. The energetic function of bitter makes it useful in treating high fevers. Aspirin is one of the oldest and most widely used substances to treat fever, pain, and headaches, and it is often used as a blood thinner. Aspirin's essential ingredient is salicylic acid, which is found in the white bark substance, essentially of a bitter composition. Goldenseal is a natural herb whose bitter component is used in treating viral and bacterial fever infections as well as the common cold. Other common bitter herbs are gentian, neem, guducci, adulsa, fenugreek, wormwood, and dandelion roots.

In excess, its use can dry out body fluids, which can lead to damaging joint stiffness and muscle aches. It can cause numbness, tremor, emaciation, and dehydration with long-term use, and it can dry out reproductive secretions. Increasing amounts can make one susceptible to vatagenic conditions.

Mental symptoms are exhibited in headache, weariness, fainting, dizziness, mental tiredness, dissatisfaction, loneliness, and cynicism.

Kashaya Rasa

Astringent taste pacifies pitta and kapha and aggravates vata in excess. It is composed mainly of the elements air and earth. Too much usage is vatagenic. Its purifying action on blood helps reduce toxic pitta. The energetic affect of cool, dry, and light assuage bodily disorders of thick mucus buildups, skin rashes, infection, and cough. It is found in tannin, haritaki, kher, alum, certain teas and coffees, unripe bananas, old honey, and pomegranates.

Many underarm deodorants have astringent properties. Be careful of aluminum addictives in deodorants. In general astringent substances are good for diarrhea as its opposing action dries. It is used in weight loss to reduce fatty tissue and water retention. It's antiseptic and anti-inflammatory actions help to cleanse and treat external skin condition. The cooling property is wonderful and beneficial to reduce heating organs and high temperatures.

In large amounts, the dry quality decreases the integrity of the mucus membrane lining the mouth, throat, and nasal passageways. This makes one prone to coughing, itchiness, and dryness. It can lead to epitaxis or nosebleeds. Overuse can weaken the integrity of the upper respiratory lining and invite viral infections. It reduces water and constricts channels (srotas) throughout the body. Chronic use interferes with the secretions of the digestive passageway. This can lead to abdominal discomfort, gastric and intestinal spasms, and flatulence. It can slow the peristalsis action in digestion and leave food in the colon longer than it should remain there. It has been used to treat chest pains, such as arrhythmia, a condition that is facilitated by high vata wind. It can lead to emaciation and loss of virility, strength, and vigor.

Mental symptoms show up as weakness, fatigue, a lack of concentration and sharpness, disorientation, spaciness, ungroundedness, and insecurity.

Diet plays an important part in influencing the doshas. Although all six tastes should be present in the meal, one can alter the ingredients to potentially correct disturbances in the body.

Management of Individual Constitution

Diseases can be categorized by an individual constitution based on the dosha type disturbance. For instance, excessive air experience on an extremely windy day can further disturbs with detrimental effect on one's vata bronchio-asthmatic condition. Because the latter is relatively vata-oriented, by increasing vata quality motion, the breath rhythm quickens, heighten anxiety and resultantly leaving the person grasping for air. Not only is the aggravated vata dosha felt physically, but it may also manifest in restlessness, nervousness, fear, and worrisome thoughts. Inversely, it has been shown that provoked mental fluctuation can spill over and manifest as neurogenic hives and skin rashes, irritable bowel syndrome, restless leg syndrome, insomnia, arrhythmia, panic attacks, and excessive blinking and tremors, and etc.

The underlying solution to treating a chronic disease is to balance the offending dosha type(s) by beginning a detoxification therapy. After the therapy, you can buildup the tissue and organ constituents by restoring a sound body constitution and resilient mind through appropriate diet. The emphasis prescribed is placed on the remedies that involve herbs, spices, foods, asanas, meditation, and lifestyle changes, all of which help cultivate strength and well-being.

East and West healing sciences ascribe to diet as the most important foundation to the prevention of disease. Ayurveda approach to the pacification of disease is to negate the doshic disturbance and restoration of it. To balance the dosha, one can ingest foods and herbs with opposing qualities to offset the antagonizing disturbance and restore the aggravated dosha. For instance, as the lightest elements of space and air, vata has qualities of rough, dry, cold, windy, light, and irregular. The approach to healing is to slow the windy, light, and dry disturbance tendencies with opposing qualities of unctuousness, moistening, warmth, fluidity, and heaviness. The energetic taste in foods best to reduce vata are sweet (heavy, liquid), sour (hot, unctuous), and salty (hot, heavy, liquid). These kapha-like attributes (warming, grounding, and stabilizing) are the opposing benefits necessary to ground vata expansiveness and bring one back to equilibrium.

The exasperation of pitta's natural qualities of heat, liquid, sharp, and intensity are given opposing substances (herbs and food) of the taste qualities of sweet (cooling), bitter (constrict), and astringent (dry) to reduce the disturbance.

The kapha type of pneumonia (there is vata and pitta types of pneumonia as well) is symptomatic of dampness, phlegm, congestion, heaviness, and shortness of breath. These kapha-related symptoms are impediments that slow the flow of oxygen in the respiratory channels and hamper the operation of the lungs. One of the five prevalent areas of kapha is the lungs. There is a sense of stuffiness and heaviness in the chest and head. Kapha is best treated with the energetic qualities of pungency, bitterness, and astringency in taste to clear and dry the obstructive channels of the nasal, throat, and lung areas.

Please note that aside from diet, the prevalent element of water is necessary for the tongue to taste the substance. The element of water is imperative to the action of taste. The substance cannot exert any action by itself in the absence of water on the tongue. Water augments the taste preceptor so that one can perceive the six tastes entering the mouth. The dehydrated person whose mouth is absolutely dry and who has wander aimlessly about in the hot desert has no taste sensation. The person wouldn't taste anything even if he or she was given food to eat. Water is an important element in treating any disease.

This concludes the chapter on ayurveda nutrition, and I cannot emphasize how important diet is to one's health enough. Ayurveda offers a way to see the properties in foods and a method to learn how one can use them to better one's health. Its approach gives one an awareness of the energetic properties of food and how these can be applied to eating styles in order to bring a sense of balance to one's life.

Chapter 12: Gunas and Foods

As mentioned earlier, the three gunas permeate every expression of consciousness in nature. It is the predominance and permutations of the guna that produces the appearance of the materialistic world as well as the psychological aspects of the mental world. Everything is represented by some aspect of the gunas—inanimate objects, insects, plants, animals, and humans. It is recognized that the intermediary source between the material world and mind, lies in food. Guna and foods play a monument part in the nourishment of the individual. The right ingredient of the guna(s) and foods make for proper digestion and the transformation into energy form that feeds the subtle constituents of the mind. Therefore, understanding of the type of food and guna quality can be one of the most profound things one can know in order to promote physical and mental well-being. So too, the unsuitable guna quality in foods can have a detrimental effect as well. Thus, foods are not just constituents but reflections of the energetic forces of the three gunas onto the physiopsychological aspects of the person.

One of the most important things one can do to change one's consciousness is to eat sattvic food and spurn bad choices of foods. The type of foods a person eats influences the individual's consciousness, and therefore, awareness is a choice in the matter. The choice to eat organic foods promotes balance to body and mental personality.

Sattvic Foods

The sattvic foods offers a healthy diet and lifestyle. Sattvic foods contain a high content of prana (life force). The essence of pranic foods feeds high index nourishment to the whole personality. It helps the body to become proficient of its physical expression in the functions of the organs down to the cellular level. One instinctively feels the nutrient effect it has on its aura. The body appears lighter and more energetic charged. The mind exudes a real sense of freshness and liveliness for the daily task and later in the day. In consummation, the change to sattvic foods reflect in the positive makeup of thoughts on the mental personality.

"As is food, so is the mind."

Sattvic foods are essentially organic, fresh, light, enjoyable to the taste, and easy to swallow and digest. Sattvic foods are unprocessed and fresh. They are organic, they naturally reflect and absorb the healing power of the cosmic rays. Sattvic foods are energetic in nature and thus recharge body and mind. They do not overstimulate or agitate the nervous, cardiac, respiratory, and digestive systems. Rather they pacify the tense mind and nerves so that the body can function better. Their wholesome content gives the body the feeling of lightness, cheerfulness, clarity, and joy. These foods are higher in pranic energy (vital life force) than other diets. The mind will feel clear and poised in calmness. One will experience better sleep, and upon awakening, the person will feed refreshed.

Sattvic (organic) foods include goat milk, buttermilk, fresh yogurt, ghee, basmati and jasmine rice, oat bran, millet, and couscous. These also include sprouted, leafy, and colorful vegetables, such as kale, green beans, asparagus, spinach, and bean sprout. There is mung bean, dahl, and lentil as well as fresh fruit juice, such as apple, pineapple, grape, pomegranate, mango, and papaya. You can also eat fruits to include dates, bananas, and melons. Raw unsalted nuts and seeds (almond, pumpkin, sunflower, walnuts, and pecan) are also healthy foods. And you can spice these foods with cumin, turmeric, saffron, mint, rosemary, cardamom, fennel, and basil. As for beverages, you can drink organic herbal teas, coffee and purified water. Drink and beverages should be taken without ice.

Rajasic Foods

Rajasic foods are stimulants that tend to bring about an increase in mental activity. The moderation in eating of rajasic foods (onion and garlic) can improve reaction times and mental acumen. Rajasic foods innate tendencies is to create motion and passion. On the negative side, the quality is associated to mutated, chemical-based, and essentially unhealthy foods that overtime drain the mind. These include the highly

Mind, Ayurveda & Yoga Psychology

charged caffeinated beverages, increased sweeten and artificial drinks, and potent energy drinks. These are basically stimulants, and sadly, they are consumed often in society. They have become very popular in today's climate. The makeup of fast foods likens to rajasic food. The inventory of the label to many of the foods on the shelves of the grocery store show noteable additives of salt and sugar to add taste and addiction, which influences the body and mind.

The sattvic foods are created by the sun, whereas rajasic foods are prepared with chemical and artificial contents. Foods that are processed, bleached, and cloned are not natural elements that can be properly digested, absorbed, and assimilated by the human digestive system.

Tamasic Foods

Tamasic foods are fermented, dry, and harder to digest. They are heavy and sluggish in nature, and they cause mind to experience drowsiness, dullness, laziness, and cloudiness. It is the worse of the three types of food to digest and absorb. Foods that are left over, stale, canned, and not fresh take on tamasic qualities. Tamasic foods include aged cheese, dark meats, shellfish, dark shades of plants like eggplant, burgers, pizza, alcohol (hard liquor), hydrogenated butter and oils, margarine, processed cereals, yogurt with fruits (different enzymes), artificial made sour cream, aged foods and too many assorted sweets. The microwaving of food causes the loss of prana energy and rescinds essential enzymes and vitamins necessary to help digestion of the ingested food. The fried and oil-based foods annul the natural freshness of them. The storage of frozen foods is away from the sun too long, and their energy suppleness is weakened over time.

Balance of the Gunas

Individuals can create harmony in their lives by balancing the qualities of the three gunas. An important goal in the practices of ayurveda and yoga is the cultivation of a sattvic lifstyle to bring about equilibrium between the physical, emotional, and mental states of the individual. The individual who seeks a sattvic lifestyle moves toward a wholesome diet, yogic postures, control of breath, concentration, meditation, positive thoughts, and good association. These people will live within their means, which reflects an equipoise relationship to themselves and the world. They will be able to handle life's surprises and daily stresses with more ease because of their clarity, calmness, and radiant outlook. They generate a more pleasant and natural lifestyle. They are positive and enjoyable to be around, and their exuberant personalities influence others in association with them.

Chapter 13: Ayurvedic Herbs for the Mind

Introduction

In this chapter we will take a look at a number of ayurveda herbs for the mind. *Medhya rasayana* are a group of herbs (ayurveda) whose primary properties are beneficial to the improvement of memory, concentration, intellect, and cognition. These medhya rasayana herbs, regularly taken, have been shown to boost immunity, longevity, and mental health. Medhya rasayana have energetic effects of tranquility, clarity, creativity, and serenity which are sattvic in nature. They contain high contents of prana that give rejuvenating energy to the mind to achieve balance. Some of the medhya rasayana herbs mentioned in this chapter include ashwagandha, brahmi, guducci, jatamunsi, jyotishmati, mandukparni, shatavari, shankhapuspi, vacha, valerian, and yashtimadu.

The science of ayurveda herbology has its origin in the ancient text of the Vedas (four volumes). The vedas mentions and classifies more than four hundred medicinal plants in three of the four volumes (two hundred ninety stated in the atharvaveda veda, eighty-one in the yajurveda veda, and sixty-seven in the rig veda). In these texts are described different types of herbal plants, the procurement and treatment of medicinal plants, the processed parts of the plant, and the exact preparation and usage of these medicinal plants. The ancient sages saw the power of the herbal plants to sustain the subtlety of health (arogya) as well as prevent and cure diseases (rogya).

Herbs for the Mind

Medhya rasayana is a specific rasayana of herbs to promote the enhancement of performance to the mind. The word *medhya rasayana* includes the two terms *medhya* (intellect) and *rasayana* (rejuvenating) respectively. It acts as a tonic therapy to improve the function of the nervous system and the brain. The energetic effect helps to improve the depths of memory, concentration, intelligence, speech, and communication, and these herbs can also widen the scope of clarity to perception.

The literal translation of *rasayana chikitsa* means "rejuvenating therapy," and its purpose is to increase ojas and promote well-being. It is one of the branches of ayurvedic medicine that focuses on longevity by delaying the aging process. Its anti-aging therapy is designed to slow down the chronological process by (1) stopping the wasting of tissues (catabolic) and (2) halting the loss of vitality.

Rasayana is a group of herbal formulas that target the seven tissues or saptu to improve each metabolic activity and produce higher ojas. The higher production and retention of ojas flows over the body and gives one brilliant skin and complexion, bright and radiant eyes, shining hair, melodious voice, cogent thought and speech, greater strength, and lucid intelligence, which supports the youthful features and workings of the physical and mental body.

In a deeper sense, the meaning of the term used to define rasayana implies the word *rasa* which is the essence, nectar, and vitality in these substance of mental herbs. *Yana* is equivalent to the particular flow (circulation) of a substance. Thus, it is the circulation of rasa or the essence of these substances that nourishes the matrix of the seven tissues and organs. By building up the function and structure of the seven tissues, rasayana helps to supplement, nourish and optimize the seven tissues. The quintessence of all seven tissues together produces the subltest energetic matter in ojas. Ojas is responsible for the overall vital energy to sustain and optimize bodily and mental health. For instance, the energetic effect of these herbs help to build cellular resistance so that one can fend off decay and the degeneration of cells. This boost to physical immunity increases constituents to respond better to bodily disturbance, and thus make the mind stronger so that one can become resilient to the encounter of daily stress.

Ashwagandha

- *Botanical name:* Withania somnifera
- *Ayurveda name:* Ashwagandha ("smell like a horse")
- *English name:* Winter Cherry

- *Rasa/Taste:* Bitter, astringent, sweet
- *Virya/Energy:* Heating
- *Vipaka/Post-digestive effect:* Sweet
- *Dosha effect:* Pacifies vata and hapha, increase pitta and ama in excess
- *Parts used:* Juice from leaves, powder, paste, roots
- *Therapeutic action:* Tonic, mental and nerve exhaustion, memory loss, insomnia, physical fatigue, general debility, giddiness, low spermatozoa, and adrenal deficiency. It is very useful for vatagenic disorders.

Ashwagandha is also known as "winter cherry." The name *ashwagandha* means "smell like a horse." It is an excellent tonic because it relaxes nervousness and mental exhaustion. It does not have a stimulating effect but rather a soothing one. Thus, it is easy to take and has no adverse effects. It is used in general debility, memory loss, decreases in muscle strength, insomnia, anxiety, and stress. It improves adrenal gland deficiency, and it is used with other herbs to treat depression, impaired neuromuscular disorder, chronic fatigue syndrome, and fibromyalgia. You can supplement bala with ashwagandha to rise from debilitating conditions of both physical and mental. The combination of bala and ashwagandha has shown to have good results to improve symptoms of fibromyalgia.

It establishes a strong immune system. As a mild aphrodisiac, it can be used to increase sexual energy. It strengthens the reproductive system and increase sexual fluid.

It has a mild sedative effect, which is helpful to settle nervousness, anxiety, tremors, and irritability. Ashwagandha oil can be topically applied to muscle cramps, spasm, pain in joints, and muscle.

Ashwagandharishta, medicated liquid concoction, is an excellent and efficient way of getting the full benefits of herbal properties without losing its potency through the digestion of the stomach. Ashwagandha has shown to be consistently effective in treating anxiety. It takes several weeks to increase concentration titrating as needed. Ashwagandha helps regulate sleep cycles, and it induces sound sleep. It can cause imaginative dreams.

Preparation: Liquid form is best. Otherwise, I would recommend 500mg capsule two to three times daily. There is no known side effect, but you should stop taking it for several days after taking for three to four weeks. This allows the body to take a break so that one doesn't grow dependent or build up a tolerance. Also, the body begins to function alone.

Bala

- *Botanical name:* Sida cordifolia
- *Ayurveda name:* Bala ("strength")
- *English name:* Indian country mallow
- *Rasa/Taste:* Sweet (madhura)
- *Virya/Energy:* Cooling

- *Vipaka/Post-digestive effect:* Sweet
- *Dosha effect:* Pacifies tridoshas but increase Ama in excess
- *Parts used:* Root, seed, stems, and leaf
- *Therapeutic action:* General tonic and useful in vatika disorders

The Sanskrit word *bala* means strength. It is one of the best rejuvenating ayurveda herbs to nourish and build the seven tissues of the body. It increases stamina, vigor, and vitality. Its tonic action strengthens the components of the neural pathways. It pacifies nerve disorders and bring them back to their strength and smoothness in transmitting neuron activities. Its grounding and stabilizing action can settle acute and mild episodes of anxiety, schizophrenia, epilepsy, and delirium. Bala's analgesic properties make it a wonderful herb to reduce vata symptoms of dull, spasm, and radiating pain (neuropathy).

Preparation: Take as a powder form of one to three grams daily. Use a medicated oil to supplement consumption.

Precaution: It has a small amount of ephedrine, which can cause concern with cardiac, hypertension, and prostate benign hypertrophy history.

Brahmi

- *Botanical name:* Centella asiatica/ Banopa monniera

- *Ayurveda name:* Brahmi
- *Rasa/Taste:* Bitter, astringent, sweet
- *Virya/Energy:* Cooling
- *Vipaka/Post digestive effect:* Sweet
- *Dosha effect:* Pacifies tridosha; vata, pitta, and kapha
- *Parts used:* Whole plant with leaves in particular and juice
- *Therapeutic action:* Tonic, mental excitation, memory loss, epilepsy, nerve exhaustion, mental fatigue, improve rate of learning, and neuralgia

Brahami leaves resemble the sulci and gyri, which make up the outer layer appearance of the brain. It is used as a brain and nerve tonic. It strengthens, regenerates, and rejuvenates brain cells. As a strong nervine tonic, it calms down the restless mind. It has a good effect on the cortex areas of brain. It helps to improve cerebral circulation and thus improve cerebral function. This can result in enhance learning, thinking, concentration, clarity, and mental alertness, and it improves memory too. It is a powerful sattvic herb that improves the faculties of the mind. It works on and supports both tarpaka (white matter) for memory and sadhaka (gray matter) for discrimination and intelligence. It works on the neurotransmitter gamma-aminobutyric acid (or gaba) to slow down the excitatory response in the brain. It has a warm and calm effect to sadhaka in the heart. Its high sattvic effect pacifies rajasic and tamasic disturbances of the mind. Its cooling property is suited to heat conditions of the head. It pacifies high vata conditions, especially connected to the nervous system. Brahmi soothe nerve cells in times of stress, fatigue, and depletion of energy.

It is an excellent rasayana herb to support the nervous system. It strengthens the structure and function of the individual nerve impulse mechanism. Studies have shown the ingredient bacosides improves nerve impulse and communication between the cells. This has shown a significant improvement to short- and long-term memory performances. Brahmi helps to support the adrenal gland. This rejuvenates the adrenal glands for times of high stress. It has been shown to reduce anxiety, panic attacks, depression, ADHD, schizophrenic, psychosis, stress, irritability, insomnia because of stress, mental fatigue, and much more. Because of its rejuvenating capacity, it is used to reverse aging in cells, and it acts as an excellent antioxidant.

Scientific studies have demonstrated brahmi beneficial in mild cases of Alzheimer's. Brahmi, harida, and ginko biloba compounds are good remedies for slowing the deteriorating actions of Alzheimer's. Brahmi, kapikacchu, and ashwagandha combined have shown good results for mild symptoms of Parkinson's disease. Brahmi, shankapushpi, jatamunsi, and vacha innate properties have people people with general nervine and brain functions. Moreover, these can be used to pacify ADHD symptoms. Always consult a physician on the usage of the aforementioned herbs, and monitor your use of ginko biloba for coagulation and potassium levels (blood level).

Preparation: Take as tablets, powder, and formulated application with brahmi ghee and saraswatirishta (liquid form).

Precaution: No major side effects have been noted; however, you should stop for a few days after lengthy usage o and then start up again.

Bhringraj

- *Botanical name:* Eclipta alba
- *Ayurveda name:* Bhringraja, Bhangra
- *Rasa/Taste:* Bitter, pungent
- *Virya/ Energy:* Heating
- *Vipaka/Post-digestive effect:* Pungent
- *Dosha effect:* Alleviates vata and kapha
- *Parts used:* Roots, leaves, seeds, and whole plant
- *System:* Nervous, plasma and blood (anemia), bone (beneficial to teeth), and marrow
- *Therapeutic action:* Nerve exhaustion, balding, hair growth and hair dye, insomnia, alleviates swelling and pain externally, enlargement of liver and spleen, and effective in various vata disorders.

Bhringraj is also known as Kehraj, which means "the king of hair." Throughout India, the oil of bringaraja is massaged into the scalp to get lustrous hair, strengthen hair follicles, promote hair growth, and avoid premature graying. It is also applied to the scalp, feet, and meridian points at bedtime to help calm the mind and produce sound and deep sleep. It can be used with other therapies to alleviate insomnia. Caraka suggests the juice of bringaraja be taken with honey to prevent the onset of senility, and it is used in rejuvenating therapies too.

Bhringraj protects the liver from toxic substances, drugs, and alcohol abuse. The root powder is used to treat cirrhosis and other liver ailments. It improves bilious flow. It alleviates vata and acts as an analgesic. It is used in disease like headache, vertigo, etc. It improves vision. It is used in night blindness and myopia. Drops of its juice is placed in eyes and ears.

Preparation: Hot and cold decoction, powder, oil, and ghee compound. Juice 6-12 ml.

Precaution: It can induce vomitting if taken in excess. Overheating will destroy its potency properties.

Calamus

- *Botanical name:* Acorns calamus linn
- *Ayurvedic name:* Vacha ("speaking")
- *English name:* Sweet Flag
- *Rasa/Tissue:* Pungent and bitter
- *Virya/ Energy:* Heating
- *Vipaka/ Post-digestive effect:* Pungent
- *Prabhav:* Medhya

- *Dosha effect:* Pacifies vata and kapha, and can irritate pitta over long term use
- *Parts used:* Rhizone and root (tuber).
- *Therapeutic action:* Vacha is a nervine (majja) and brain tonic, medhya, and rejuvenating herb. It is a medhya tonic for both nerves and the brain. Its expansive action increases circulation and oxygen intake, and it improves thinking, learning, and higher cognition function. It has been used to counteract spasms, chronic sinus infections, and bodily pain. Being analgesic and anti-inflammatory, its paste is useful in rheumatoid arthritis, and painful joints.

Calamus works to clear toxins of both majjavaha (nerve channels) srotas and manovaha (mental channels) srotas. This results in better circulation to the deep tissue areas of the brain and central nervous system. It is a brain tonic that promotes better concentration, clarity, self-awareness, memory, and intelligence. It improves cognitive skills and reaction time by synchronizing the two cortexes of the brain.

The Sanskrit meaning of the word *vacha* is to increase the power of speech. It improves speech so that one can express internal thoughts. It reduces mental stagnation by stimulating the faculties of the brain. It allows better communication to thoughts and feelings. It helps to expand self-awareness in relationship to others.

Calamus steadies the mind of disturbances to stress, headache, dizziness, lethargy, fear, seizures, shock, convulsion, mania, and mental congestion. It pacifies the negative tendencies of sadness, grief, irritation, mental stress, anxiety, hysteria, and depression. It rapidly clears sinus conditions and thus affects the physiological passageway to the brain. It is used to treat the neurological disorders of neuralgia, spasmodic episodes, epilepsy (medicated ghee), shock, and seizures.

Useful in alleviating vata and kapha of the respiratory tract. It is used extensively in cough, asthma, pharyngitis, and laryngitis. Vacha lozenges is useful in the mouth to sooth irritation of the former condtions.

Calamus helps to balance disturbed tamoguna by clearing kapha congestion from manovaha strota. This can lead to greater awareness of consciousness. It helps to clear stagnated emotions. It is used in conjunction with shankapusphi, brahmi, and jatamunsi to reduce ADHD symptoms.

Medicated calamus with ghee is beneficial for various mind applications, including exhaustion and cloudiness. Small amount of the powder with honey can be given to children (one year and older). Consult an ayurveda physician first for the latter and other recommendations before you attempt to use it.

Preparation: medicated ghee, suggest 250–300mg once or twice daily, milk decoction, and capsules form. Its juice is used as ear drops for earache and tinnitus.

Precaution: High doses should not be used for lengthy periods. Epitaxis (nosebleeds) can occur with abuse. Calamus can be sniffed to relieve acute and chronic sinus conditions. It tends to work rather quickly. High dosages can cause vomiting. It can have an addictive effect, and use should be monitored.

Guduchi

- *Botanical name:* Tinospora cordifolia
- *Ayurveda name:* Gudwel, amrita, and guducci ("one which protects the body)
- *Rasa/Taste:* Bitter, astringent, sweet
- *Virya/Energy:* Heating
- *Vipaka/Post-digestive effect:* Sweet
- *Dosha effect:* Pacifies all doshas; wonderful medhya herb to reduce high pitta
- *Parts used:* The whole plant is used, especially bark. The fresh part of the guduchi plant is more therapeutic than dry part.
- *Therapeutic action:* Pacify high pitta, rejuvenator of mind, opens mind srota (channel), good for general debility, rasayana for all seven dhatus. It is useful in a number of skin disorders – along with neem, haridra, guggulu, khadir and amla. Externally oil applied to pacify dermatoses, gout, erysepalas, burning and irritating sensation due to its anti-heating effect (pitta). Juice of guducci is good for chronic fever, malaria and typhoid fever.

Guduchi is a sattvic herb that promotes calmness and purity of cellular function and mind. It is a powerful medhya (mind) rasayana that strengthens and broadens the capacity of the mind. It opens the emotional heart. It promotes clarity in thinking and expression. It is a potent tonic and rejuvenates ojas and the immune system. The herb binds and removes amavisha (internal toxins from body and mind). It relieves high heat (pitta) in the body. It is useful in purifying and detoxifying impurities in the blood whose acidic contents can cause headaches, migraines, and mental fatigue.

People who consume alcohol benefit from guduchi treatment because of its beneficial effect in regenerating liver tissue. You can increase the potency of this herbal effort by stopping or limiting your alcohol intake.

Preparation: Extract, powder of 250–500mg twice day.

Precaution: No significant side effects have been found.

Jatamunsi

- *Botanical name:* Nordostachys jatamansi
- *Ayurveda name:* Jatamunsi
- *English name:* Indian spikenard, valeman
- *Rasa/Taste:* Sweet, bitter and astringent
- *Virya/Energy:* Cooling
- *Vipaka/Post-digestive energy:* Pungent
- *Prabhav:* Bhutaghna and manosrotaghna
- *Dosha effect:* Reduces high vatagenic conditions by snigdha (oily) action, pittagenic conditions by cooling, bitter, astringent, and

sweet properties, and kaphagenic conditions by bitter and penetrating properties: tridosha action
- *Parts used:* Roots, freash powder are used
- *Therapeutic action:* Mild sedative, circulatory, skin (paste), urinary, nervine and brain tonic (manasaroga), its act primarily on the nervous system

Jatamunsi is a bhutaghna herb whose specific action is to calm and relax brain activity. It promotes good mental health. The rejuvenative properties of jatamunsi are helpful in the management of anxiety, depression, hysteria, schizophrenia, epilepsy, agitation, and mental exhaustion. It pacifies high-stress vatagenic disorders, nervous headaches, fear, tremors, and convulsions. It has been shown to relieve heart palpitations and angina. It induces deep sleep without drowsiness upon awaken.

Jatamansi is very effective headache, hypertension, cough, dyspnea, analgesic (oil to skin), and stimulates kidney to improve micturition, dysuria, and cystitis, and whose tonic action is good for general weakness.

Preparation: Take 250–500mg twice daily. Take one tablespoon of fresh jatamunsi powder with warm milk.

Precaution: Prolonged and high dosages can cause hyperemesis and stomach-gripping

Sensations, and dysentery.

Joytishmati

- *Botanical name:* Celastrus paniculatus
- *Ayurveda name:* Joytishmati kula
- *English name:* Staff tree
- *Rasa/Taste:* Pungent and bitter
- *Virya/Energy:* Heating
- *Vipaka/Post-digestive effect:* Pungent
- *Prabhava:* Medhya, improves intellect vitality

Dosha effect: Balances vata and kapha but its hot potency can aggravate pitta in long term use

- *Parts used:* Leave, seed, and oil
- *Therapuetic effect:* Nervine, brain tonic, neuroprotective, sedative, nootropic in activity, and improves memory by medhya action. It promotes intelligence, sadhakagni (sharp agni) increases the grey matter of brain (pitta) that sharpens intelligence and discrimination.

Joytishmati is a rejuvenating herb with specific effects on the mind. It stimulates intelligence capacity, and it improves memory and concentration. It can be used as an antidepressant, and it calms a restless mind or headache. It also promotes sound sleep. It stimulates the heart and improves cardiac output (bradycardia). Its nasya application is good for asthma and bronchitis. External use is excellent for soothing vatagenic conditions. Thus, application to conditions of backache, sciatica, and arthritis.

Preparation: Medicated nasya oil treatment of two to four drops twice daily. Seed powder of 250–500mg twice daily.

Precaution: It can induce vomiting if taken in excess.

Shankapushpi

- *Botanical name:* Foeniculum vulgare gaertn
- *Ayurveda name:* Shankapushpi
- *English name:* Shankapushpi
- *Rasa/Taste:* Sweet, bitter and astringent
- *Virya/Energy:* Cooling
- *Vipaka/Post-digestive effect:* Sweet
- *Prabhav:* Medhya rasayana (specific for mind)
- *Dosha effect:* Pacifies vata, pitta and kapha = especially vatapittashamak
- *Parts used:* Plant, juice, seeds
- *Therapeutic action:* Mental exhaustion, lack of concentration, cloudy and sluggish thinking, memory loss, and fatigue.

Shankapushpi's flowers resemble the shanka or conch shell. Its use is for mental clarity and concentration. Its relaxing effect pacifies anxiety, fear, depression, phobias, mental fatigue, emotional exhaustion, stress, manic phase, post-traumatic disorders, and insomnia (bedtime). It has shown good results in treating ADHA in formula of brahmi, jatamansi, vacha and licorice. It can clear the mind and improve concentration. It is a rejuvenating herb for mind and nerve tissue. Is is also used in distension, pain in abdomen, dysentery and piles.

Preparation: Suggested amount of powder 250–500mg twice daily. 2-4 oil drops

Precaution: There are no adverse effects.

Shatavari

- *Botanical name:* Asparagus racemosus
- *Ayurveda name:* Shatavari ("hundred husbands")
- *English name:* Wild Asparagus
- *Rasa/Taste:* Sweet and bitter
- *Virya/Energy:* Cooling
- *Vipalca/ Post-digestive effect:* Sweet
- *Dosha effect:* Balances vata and pitta, and can aggravate kapha with similar attributes of sweet and cool on long-term use
- *Parts used:* Tuber
- *Therapeutic effect:* Rejuvenating herb for female reproduction system, mild aphrodisiac, sattvic properties, and nutritive tonic for rasa and rakta dhatu, the latter to alleviate bleeding disorders, and cardiotonic effect. It gives energy to brain and nerves, and reduces syncope disorder.

Shatavari is a rejuvenating herb. The rasa energetic effect helps with the circulation of nourishment to the vital organs. Shatavari property is sattvic and thus increases ojas. Its cooling nature calms down heated mental emotion states.

It cools and cleanses high pitta toxins from blood. Its cooling effect reduces high sadhaka pitta, which is responsible for discrimination of thoughts and reason. It works to reduce pulsating headaches, overworked thinking, and high fevers of unknown origins.

It promotes healthy hormone balance. It is considered one of the best rasayana to support and strengthen the female reproductive tissues. It is useful in menopause conditions to treat hot flashes, low libido, cramps, excessive bleeding, increase lactation, sexual secretion, and infertility. It can act as a mild aphrodisiac in male impotence and low sexual energy.

Preparation: Take a capsule and in powder form of 250–500mg twice daily, and juice with honey is good for shortness of breath.

Precaution: There are no adverse effects because of its diuretic effect.

Tagra (Valerian)

- *Botanical name:* Valeriana wallichi Dc.
- *Ayurvedic Name:* Tagara
- *English name:* Indian valerian
- *Rasa:* Pungent, bitter
- *Virya energy:* Heating
- *Vipaka:* Pungent
- *Dosha effect:* Pacifies vata and kapha; and pitta in smaller amounts.

- *Parts used:* Root contains volatile oil; yellow and bitter substance, and rhizome part
- *Therapeutic action:* Nervine, mental exhaustion, anxiety, sedative, calmative, anticonvulsant, antispasmodic in pain, hypnotic for insomnia.

Valerian (tagra) is a calming herb that soothes the nervous system quickly without the drowsiness effect of the Western equivalent. Tagara, the Indian type, is tolerated well by the stomach (unlike its Western counterpart). It works on the central and automatic nervous system. It relaxes sympathetic states of high nerve excitement associated in anxiety-related disorders. Dosages of 200 to 400mg daily has been shown to be effective in calming nerves. It is analgesic, and it relaxes the mind too. Furthermore, it is useful in mental and physical exhaustion, emotional stress, panic attacks, headaches, migraines, anxiousness, and restlessness. It is a wonderfully relaxing herb that has shown to be effective in treating insomnia. It puts you to sleep gradually. It provides sound sleep without drowsiness upon awaken. Like with any herb, it should be taken five to six days a week, and one should take one to two days off. This allows the body to react to its natural safety mechanism and regulate tolerance level. Because of its strong antispasmodic action, it is used for chronic pain, that reduces bodily discomfort and anxiety. It is used to treat menstrual cramping. So too, when combine with shankapushpi, brahmi, and vacha it can be used to treat ADHD. It is useful in cardiac arrhythmias and hepatoprotective in action.

It is one of the most important ayurveda herbs to reduce anxiety, insomnia, menopause, and stress. One should seek consultation by an ayuredic physician before using it.

Preparation: Recommend powder of 250–500mg form twice daily as needed. Also tincture and infusion formula.

Precaution: It should not be taken during pregnancy and breast-feeding. Not to be given to children. It can be addictive, and one can grow dependent with long-term use. Short-term use is recommended. Overdose can cause fainting, vomiting, and headaches, and can induce sleep in some.

Yashti Madhu—Licorice

- *Botanical name:* Glycerrhiza glabra Linn.
- *Ayurveda name:* Yashti Madhu
- *English name:* Liquorice
- *Rasa/Taste:* Sweet
- *Virya/Energy:* Cooling
- *Vipaka/Post-digestive effect:* Sweet
- *Dosha effect:* Pacifies vata and pitta conditions. It can aggravate kapha conditions in long trm usage. It is a natural steroid. It increases water retention and potassium level to rise.
- *Parts used:* root
- *Therapeutic action:* Spasmolytic, nutritive, livotonic, expectorant, alterative, demulcent, anti-inflammatory, gives strength to nerves

Dr. John Cosby

Licorice is a sweet-tasting herb that gives satisfaction to the mind. It is a brain tonic that is effective in reducing overheated thinking. It is an exoogenous sustabance to secrete cortisol concentrations and respond to anti-inflammation, asthma, bronchospasm, hyperacidity, shingles, psoriasis, and eczema conditions. It is homeostatic and purifies blood (rakta dhatu). Its diuretic action helps in micturition and dysuria. It increases sperm count and premature ejaculation (mix ghee, milk and honey). Apply to skin disorders that are burning, irritating, itchy, as well as, smooth complexion to the face (face pack)

Ayurveda recognizes licorice to be an important herb used to treat inflammatory throat and lungs symptoms. It is an expectorant and helpful in hoaseness of voice, cough, tuberculosis, and fever. It indirectly affects the subdosha energies of udana, avalambhaka, tarpaka, and sadhaka, which governs self-expression, speech, feeling, memory, and intelligence.

Preparation: A powder form of 250–500mg twice daily is suggested. Formulation in Yashtyadipak and Yashtimadhvadi taila.

Precaution: As a natural corticosterone, it can affect kapha to retain water and gain weight. Long-term use causes high blood pressure, and thus, individuals with high pitta should avoid long term usage. It can become emetic if given in excess.

Chapter 14: Asanas for Vata, Pitta, and Kapha Constitutions

Introduction

In addition to dietary measures, yoga asanas can be a powerful tool for restoring balance to a person's physical constitution. The yogic tradition specifically came to recognize that there were certain asanas that were particularly useful for different constitutions. In this chapter we will look at what asanas are most beneficial to a person's particular constitution.

Yoga for Vata

Asana postures center on counterbalance to space and air. The focus of yoga asanas for the vata type is generally done in a quiet atmospheric space (preferably in a small class with less distractions) as well as steady and repetitive postures (making it easy to focus). The hip and seat positions are good for their grounding effects. The regular practice of vata postures will have a gentle and easy flow so that one can be attentive, composed and consistent in the postures.

As the vata person ages, his or her restless tendency shows in joint stiffness, spasm, backache, body ache, tension, and achy headache. The exasperated vata type has difficulty staying still and holding posture with any length of time. Intense and strenuous movements cause distraction and restlessness, both which tend to remove the mind from the gain of steadiness and comfort to the physical postures done.

Asana Postures for Vata

Vata types in general are drawn to constant change because of their primary composition of air and space. Yoga is a strong tool to steady and calm the flow of that constant movement. The yoga disciplines strengthen mental focus and concentration. The benefit of focus allows the vata person to hold postures for longer periods of time. As mentioned, sitting poses geared toward the pelvic and lower abdomen areas are extremely good. Kapha type yoga postures are recommended to oppose the light and mobile qualities of the vata person. Regular practice is important to maintain uniformity and the expected outcome to the postures (familiarity with less distraction). The vata types can be easily agitated by factors of stress, cold weather, long hours, fatigue, and missed meals, which exasperates them into restlessness, nervousness, and wandering thoughts. Remember that the tridoshas exist in everyone but in different degrees, and each of the dosha types are dominant at some point in the day and life.

Before practicing yoga asanas, one can do alternate nostril breathing to calm the mind. The mind controls the body!

Mind, Ayurveda & Yoga Psychology

Yoga Asanas for Vata Disturbances of Anxiety

There are many disturbances to the exasperated vata type, but in this book we will only explore the condition of anxiety, as it is very common in the general population, not only to the vata person.

Anxiety

- Padangstasana—forward bend pose (oxygenates blood to head).
- Deviasana—goddess pose (empowers you).
- Shavasana—corpse pose (release thought, emotion, feeling, and tightness).
- Ardha Matsyendrasana—half twist pose (strengthen the spine, and floor posture).
- Sukasana—easy pose (relieve exhaustion, and promotes peace and calm).
- Garudasana—eagle pose (improve concentration).
- Vaishistasana—side plank pose (settles mind, concentration).
- Tadasana—mountain pose (improves body balance and grounds the mind).
- Yoga Nidra—deep sleep experience, (good for stress relief).
- Vajrasana—thunderbolt pose (stabilize mind, strengthens spine and nerve).
- Virabhadrasana—warrior pose (invigorates respiratory and circulatory, increases strength and flexibility to muscles).

If you are unfamiliar with these postures, it is best to attend a local yoga class, and you can also expose yourself to the different asana postures with a DVD recording. It is best to start with a yoga instructor to eliminate bad habits before beginning the recording in your home. The practice of yoga for the vata person should not be done before bedtime (except for nidra yoga).

Yoga for Pitta

This focuses on the principle of fire and water. These people are strong-minded and feel the need to complete all of the attempted postures. Their competitive nature forces them to be perfectionists in yoga postures, and thus, they demand more of themselves. They generate high heating energy in the achievement of each posture. When out of balance, their arrogance and ego will push them beyond to finish all asanas in a timely manner. The pitta person does not know how to say no and poses a risk to themselves in the form of physical injury. They will try to work through joint pain and muscle tightness to complete the entirety of postures. Pitta's natural tendencies to body heat and emotions should begin with gentle pranayama exercises. They are attracted to the challenge of advanced yoga practices like astanga yoga. They are of strong or medium build with good muscle tone and therefore enjoy the physical endurance of such yoga strengthening practices. No challenge is big enough for them. Not perfecting the asana postures can result in frustration and irritability. Headstrong pitta types can manifest in physical pain, inflammation, strain, stiffness, and hurting joints by pushing themselves too far to reach perfection.

Their competitive nature often makes them critical of themselves and the instructor. Ironically, pitta individuals tend to become excellent yoga instructors.

Asana Postures for Pitta

They tend to be thinkers and detailed. The perfectionist approach makes them want to master all of the postures, but they can develop "insensitivity" to the real reason for doing yoga asana. Their minds take over the mechanics of asana posture instead to attuning and listening to the inner quietness of the full postures. Yoga teaches the person to become sensitive, flexible, relaxed, patient, and humble in order to develop the mind. An important posture for pitta person to quiet the mind is in the resting period between the asana postures, the corpse position. This inactive posture allows the body and mind to cool and settle down after the finished postures. The pitta person will think the rest period is a waste of time and instead want to move onto the next posture.

In conjunction to asana, bring awareness so that your breath rhythm is smooth, gentle, and slow during the entire motion of the posture.

Pitta yoga asanas helps to relieve fiery emotions, fatigue, exhaustion, and anger.

- Garbasana—child pose (improve mood).
- Shavasana—corpse pose (release thought, emotion, feeling, and tightness).
- Jnanansa—mental discipline (focus mind).
- Bhairavasana—series of advance postures (letting go).
- Marjariasana—cats pose (stretches spinal cord which strengthen nerves and reduces tension).
- Sukhasana—easy pose (inner joy and happiness).
- Parighasana—gate pose (stabilize mind).
- Parsvottanasana—pyramid/intense stretch pose (nonjudgmental).
- Trikonasana—triangle pose (strengthens neck muscle, relieves neck pain and trunk tension).
- Bhujangasana—cobra pose (stretches entire spine, strengthen nerve, and releases muscular back tension).
- Anjaneyasana—low lung pose (synchronize breath).

The following postures are helpful to relieve pitta headaches, which tend to be throbbing and pulsating.

- Apanasana—knee to chest (calm breath and center mind).
- Shavasana—corpse pose (release thought, emotions, feelings, and tightness).
- Matsyasana—fish pose (works facial and neck tension).

- Padma—lotus pose (settle body).
- Pavamuktasana—wind releasing pose (improve circulation, free tension to neck and back).
- Uttanasana—stand forward pose (relieves stress, fatigue, head tension).
- Yoga nidra—deep sleep-like experience (stress relief to entire body).
- Trikonasana—triangle pose (strengthens neck muscle, relieves neck tension).
- Bhujangasana—cobra pose (stretch entire spine, releases muscular back tension).
- Vajrasana—thunderbolt pose (stabilize mind, strengthen spine and nerve).
- Sarvangasana—shoulder stand pose (relief of headache, improve cerebral circulation)

Before undertaking any asana posture, you should discuss your safety with a yoga instructor and your medical physician.

Yoga for Kapha

Physical attributes are representative of earth and water, the heaviest of elements. The solid and dense elements make for a strong, sturdy, and powerful base. Their firm base tends to allow for steady attention, strong stamina, and ease to hold poses for longer periods. The liquid element gives natural lubrication to joints and help them get into poses more easily. Water and earth characteristics naturally connect them to

Mother Earth, which is the platform that asanas are done on. Because the seat of kapha is the stomach and the lung characteristics of fluid and elasticity, asanas should focus more on abdomen and chest poses to restore balance. The kapha individual, when motivated to practice the yoga postures, will benefit more with visualization and breathing exercises.

Asanas for Kapha

When out of balance, their attributes of slow, cold, dense, liquid, and dull make them vulnerable to states of laziness, sluggishness, and lethargy, and they can easily build up fat and watery substances. Their large body types impose low motivation as they hang onto old emotions, and they often lack the will to change. During yoga exercises, they need to be encouraged because they are comfortable with doing the least amount of effort. They need to move out of false complacency. They tend to be attracted to hatha yoga rather than the more intense yogic systems. Yoga sessions need to be supplemented with other tools to assist with poses. An important means is the practice of stimulating pranayama exercises to energize and expand the mind.

Just as respiratory ailments can cause nasal and chest congestion, stagnant emotions of the mind can cause lethargy and cloudiness in thinking. When balanced, kapha individuals are wonderfully patient, compassionate, loving, caring, and giving to others.

Yoga Asanas for Kapha Mental Disturbance for Depression

Depression

- Halasana—plough poses (helps to reduce sluggishness, lethargy, and dullness).
- Paschimottanasana—seated forward bend pose (focuses mind, relieve stress, and mild depression).
- Ardha Chandrasana—half moon pose (reduces fatigue and anxiety).
- Shavasana—corpse pose (releases thought, feeling, emotions, and tightness).
- Tarasana—star pose (helps with energy, strengthens lung and chest).
- Virabhadrasana—warrior pose (strengthen body).
- Shastankasana—hare pose (increase blood to head).
- Surya Namaskana—salute to the sun (improve concentration, and stabilizes mind).
- Mayurasana—peacock (grace in balance, and improves concentration).
- Uttanasana—intense stretch pose (calm brain, reduce stress, mild depression).
- Simhasana—lion pose (invigorates, opens chest, moves air in lungs).
- Apanasana—knee to chest pose (stimulate nerves, and calms the mind).

Dr. John Cosby

Most yogic asanas are beneficial in that they invigorate and strengthen the three dosha types. There are exceptions to doing certain asanas, such as head stand posture that is contraindicated to high pitta condition. The yoga instructor should be informed of any limitation before the start of asanas class. Notify the instructor of any bodily heart conditions. Never attempt to start on your own without proper guidance because asanas can be constraining and exhausting at first. In doing yoga, one should relax and feel comfortable doing each posture and not feel in any pain. The beautiful thing about yoga is any age or person can do many of the postures, as asanas can be modified to fit anyone's physical limitations.

Yoga establishments that have been around for years tend to portray authenticity to the principles and practices of yoga asansa. Look for the certification of the instructors. You can also speak with your medical physician about any concerns in self limited medical conditions.

Yoga has become more mainstream in our society which has caught the attention of physicians.

Consult an Ayurvedic Physician

If you have chronic health issues, consult an ayurvedic physician. Or consider going to an ayurvedic retreat center that includes pancha karma treatment along with yoga and meditation. You should not begin yoga postures on your own unless given instructions by someone knowledgeable of the many postures.

Part 4: Integrating the Yoga Traditions

Chapter 15: Karma, Bhakti, Raja, and Jnana Yogas

Yoga sees the individual as a whole being and spiritual personality. It recognizes that people have the potential to live out their true identities. By comparison, many of us see ourselves lacking in an integral personality. We are reminded of this in our day-to-day experiences of negative traits that show up unannounced (e.g., the rise of anger, doubt, confusion, indolence, dullness, fear, anxiety, and mistaken notions of illusion, instability, and distracted thoughts waves formed by our operating mind) as well as the physical manifestation of palpitation, panic attacks, and migraine headaches. We feel overwhelmed by them and not in control of these rising partial thoughts and habitual happenings, and we are left with the feeling of being isolated, helpless, and subservient to unnatural conditions of life.

Yoga is a science of spiritual psychology that gives one deep insight into the workings of the mind. The principles of yogi philosophy are a combination of an assortment of teaching methods to uncover the potentiality of the mind. On a practical level, the aspiring yogi becomes his or her own psychoanalyst in exploring and uncovering the plethora of layers in the mind. A deeper study of the mind gives a clearer insight into the reoccurrence of events and circumstances that do not happen by accident or chance but are the by-product of past thoughts and actions played out in the present conditions. Yoga recognizes the present conditions can be negated or sublimated by realizing you have the ability to change the pattern of your mind and your negative thought to positive ones, which changes your perception and the way you react to the setting of characters and situations in your life. You have the endurance to overcome all adversities and harsh conditions and be free of them. Every development in life has a meaning and significance that is to be learned with appropriate insightfulness. You are the navigator of your destiny. The beauty of yoga psychology is it does not depend on who you are or what you are doing to create transformation in your life.

Yoga classifies the mind in three planes of consciousness—the unconscious, conscious, and super-conscious. Each of these consciousnesses is not a separate entity from one another, but rather together, they make up the workings of the human personality. The unconscious plane is the storage of all past lives and impressions accumulated over time by the conscious mind. The unconscious is where the karmic impressions of one's many lives are held. They lay low until triggered by some external stimuli on the surface of the conscious level and then come into action. The unconscious plane regurgitates these deep-rooted impressions back into the world when one needs to respond and perform some action by the conscious mind. At the surface level, most people are unaware of these rising impressions that impose their dominance and direction on our minds. The unawareness of these impressions can cause irritability, fear, anger, and confusion that are played out in life without any understanding to the association of these hidden expressions of the unconscious mind. Yoga recognizes that for many of us, the irregularities that appear in our personalities stem from the driving force of the unconscious and subconscious onto the awaken mind. Thus, the unconscious mind left without awareness can dictate behavior patterns to shape and form our personalities.

In *Applied Yoga,* Swami Jyotirmayanda states the superconscious mind is the intuitive mind in man. When the unconscious mind is freed from the impressions of complexes and negative karmas, it gives way to the functioning of the purest state of mind—which is luminous, expansive, and transparency. It is through this state of mind that one realizes oneself to be different from the egoistic personality of day to day life, burdened with perishable problems; one realizes oneself to be Supreme Self—eternal, immortal, and infinite.

Yoga gives a scientific and practical understanding on how to change your unconscious in terms of adjusting the operational mechanism of the conscious psyche. One can become aware (1) unconscious being the recipient to the by-product of thought being acted out by the awaken person. One also has the ability to change the mechanism in the thinking pattern of the active mind. By changing one's perception, one could alter the quality of the perceived object and its meaning.

Dr. John Cosby

On a relative level, the perceived content of an object is seen differently by the perception of many minds seeing the same object through their own eyes. For example, one sees the rope as a snake in the dark and is overwhelmed by fear over the imaginary and unreal object. Another person sees the rope with dullness and is confounded and slow to react. The person does not know whether to stay or run away. The third person sees the rope as a rope with clarity and thus sees the perceived object as it is. The content in all three cases is identical, but it is perceived differently because they are not the same minds. Thus, the range of clarity, uncertainty, and delusion shapes how one perceives an object and the particular meaning associated to it.

The Many Systems of Yogic Philosophy

The many systems of yogic philosophy give us deeper teaching and practical disciplines necessary to remove the impurities in our personalities into integrating ones. All of the yogic practices are driven to raise the energetic life-form of prana and sattva qualities within the body and mind. This can be accomplished through eating organic foods, good conducts of behavior, regular exercises, regulating breath, positive thinking, good association, study of sacred scriptures, meditation, devotion to higher being, and selfless service to others who are less fortunate.

One should learn the art of self enquiry into the limitation and conditions we have self-imposed on our psyches. For many the world is filled with adversity and negativity, which block freedom of expression. By witnessing our minds can one gain insight into how thoughts fall under the negative influence that appear to arise unprompted in our heads. Rajas characteristics that are impure (passion, activity, restlessness, vanity, greed, lust, self-centeredness, and insatiable possession of materials) can bind one's mind by affixating attention on objects that leave little room for other thoughts. The increasing disturbance of the raja's mind becomes more concerned with the processes of the materialistic world, thus leaving the core of the inner personality to expressing its true self. The increasing tamas characteristics of inertia, heaviness, dullness, deceit, insensitivity, and slowness produces greater crystallization patterns of thoughts, which can delay the response to decision making and/or obstruct our natural flow in the thinking process of clarity.

By removing the impurities of rajas and tamas, one's personality becomes more sattvic in qualities - purity, brilliance, transparency and serenity. The predominance of luminosity and tranquility sublimate the negativity of rajas and tamas, and bestows the positivity of sattvic vibration on one's mind-set.

Integral Yoga

In his book Applied Yoga, Swami Jyotirmayananda states, every human being has four aspects in his personality—Reason, Will, Emotion and Action.

The integration of one's personality depends upon a balanced and harmonious development of these aspects. The Yoga-process is one's integral process, but named differently accordingly to its specialized emphasis. The Yoga that trains reason is known as Jnana Yoga or Yoga of Wisdom. The Yoga that develops blazing love of God and causes emotional integration is called Bhakti Yoga or Yoga of Devotion. The Yoga that enables one to control the mind through meditation is called Raja Yoga. The Yoga that enables one to prepare his psychological being to face and confront the day-to-day activities of life, and also unfolds his hidden potentialities is called Karma Yoga, the Yoga of Action. These four aspects of Yoga—right reasoning, true willing, love of higher being, and right activity are not opposed to each other, but rather, are four aspects of one integral movement towards life's ascending heights. There are many branches and sub-branches of these four Great Yogas. For example, Hatha Yoga, the yoga of physical poses and exercises is only a branch of Raja Yoga (Patanjali third limb) – the Yoga of Asanas.

To paraphrase, karma yoga allows you to develop loving thoughts so that you can embrace truth and perform your selfless duty to others and society. Bhakti yoga allows you to fine-tune feelings, purify your highest love in your heart, and bring about transcendental feelings into your personality. Jnana yoga clears and refines your intellect and reason through the sacred teachings so that you can the rise in intuitive wisdom, and raja yoga cultivates the power of will, concentration, and meditation for the mastery of mind, unlocking the doors of enlightenment. The four yogas are not separate or antagonistic to one another but rather complementary parts for the integration of the spiritual personality.

Just as different body parts come together to form the overall physical structure and function of the human organism, the movement of integral yoga emphasizes the blending of the main aspects of the mind in reason, feeling, will, and action, to help one another work toward integrating the whole personality.

The Four Major Yogas

1. *Karma yoga* is "yoga of action, purification." Karma yoga recognizes that everything we do is based on action. Every action must be accompanied with a righteous attitude, motivation, and commitment so that you can perform whatever your duty or dharma is and to give the selfless fruit of action to the supreme being. One's duty is neither inferior nor superior, but rather it is a truthful experience of selfless service to the suffering of humanity. Karma yoga is doing virtuous deeds without expecting anything in return. It is the abandonment of fruitful expectation of gaining fame, wealth, and ownership. It is the movement to perform selfless duties for others and the community. Karma yoga is the cultivation of the

psychological aspects of the mind so that one can carry out selfless action with the understanding that the whole world is the manifestation of the omnipresent being. Every day's activity is served with the constant remembrance of the eternal being. The selfless act to service humanity with bhavana (pure feeling) leads to the purification of the heart. Karma yoga is the first step on the journey path to God. Karma yoga purifies the feelings in the heart of a bhakti yogi to develop unconditional love of higher being. Loving devotion purifies the heart center to transform reason and intelligence into intuitive knowledge (jnana yoga). Pure heart, devotion, and intuitive intelligence help one master raja yoga in dharana (concentration) and dhyana (meditation) in order to experience the super-conscious state of samadhi.

2. *Bhakti yoga* is the path that leads to the transcendental feeling of pure love and devotion, allowing one to fully surrender to the supreme being or Krishna. The Sanskrit word bhakti is derived from the root bhaj, which literally translates as "to be attached to God." It is the worship between the beloved deity and the loving devotee. The transcending relationship between the two cultivates unconditional love, sweetness, and adoration toward the omnipresent. The objective form of the deities leads the person to a higher plane of unconditional love. The sprout

Mind, Ayurveda & Yoga Psychology

of unconditional love causes one to lose his or her individuality by melting into the sweetness of the unmanifested. There is no separation between the two, and nothing else matters in the world.

a. Bhakti yoga helps a person become humble because it teaches how to service without selfish motives. Devotional service to the Lord or Krishna can also put an end to all sinful activities. Bhakti worship can help a person eliminate conditional sin or karma and wash the heart of negative emotions, such as jealousy, hatred, greed, anger, malice, among other, and accept divinity expressions of joy, compassion, peace, bliss, and love. Once sinful activities have stopped, a person no longer receives sinful reaction, which leads to a peaceful mind.

b. In a peaceful state of mind, a person can understand transcendental knowledge, which leads to spiritual vision. As spiritual vision increases, the heart opens further to higher unconditional love, and the mind intensifies in intuitive knowledge, which spontaneously guides one on how to live in this world and not be affected by kama (desire) and karma (action).

3. *Rajas yoga* is synonymous with "king among yoga," "royal yoga," "yoga of the mind", and

"ashtanga yoga." It is the yoga path associated with specific disciplines but practical to the mastery development of the mind. In the commentaries of the Patanjali yoga sutras, there are the eight limbs of ashtanga yoga, discussed in chapter 5. The primary objective of ashtanga yoga is the cultivation of the mind through a series of practical steps to control the cessation of any modification in thought waves. By removing distracted thoughts, the mind is left to experience quiet and clarity, which fosters spontaneity and intuitive reasons in interacting with the self, others, and surroundings. The ongoing progression of intuitive knowledge refines one so that he or she can attain the subtle state of self-realization.

4. *Jnana yoga* is the path of wisdom. It uses the intellect to ascend the ladder to higher consciousness. The intellect is a tool we can use to explore deeper into the understanding of our true identities. The intellect is a means that one must eventually go beyond in order to realize the self. The intellect must not be confused with mathematics, language, and scientific knowledge. It is the use of the mind to unfold its intrinsic potential and to rise in spontaneous thinking, clarity, precision in perception, astuteness, and reason. The purpose of jnana yoga is to acquire intuitive knowledge through the progressive understanding of the sacred scriptures (reflected inward of our self),

the ability to listen and reflect on the guru's words to the mystic knowledge of the sages and saints, the advance in singular concentration and contemplative meditation, and the endurance in self-inquiry to the universal question, "Who am I?" To take up the movement of jnana yoga, one must acquire a clear understanding of the four qualifications of viveka, vairagya, shat-sampat and mumukshutva.

a. *Viveka* is the subtle ability to differentiate the permanent and transient aspects in the creative world. The end process is the nature of permanency or the eternal, the absolute self alone. By repeated effort and inquiry, one develops an instinctive awareness of the separation of what is real and unreal, changing and unchanging, and right and wrong. The discriminatory aspect of the intellect enables one to recognize objectivity is not real but rather sequential and linked to time and space.

b. *Vairagya* or dispassion is the progressive development of inner strength of mind to turn away from the enjoyable sensory objects (bhoga). The practice of vairagya enables the mind to become disengage with the craving senses and the dependency on the objective world. Dispassion opposes the imaginary and transient gratification of the world. Intead, one can develop real and permanent enjoyments of life.

c. *Shat-Sampat* is the implementation of the six qualities necessary to progress up the rungs of consciousness. These six virtuous qualities are sama (serenity), dama (control over the senses), uparati (lack of selfishness), titiksha (ensurance and tolerance), shraddha (faith), and samadhana (mental balance).

d. *Mumukshutva* is the burning or intense desire for liberation or moksha.

Integral yoga blends other minor yoga (hatha yoga, mantra yoga, japa yoga, kundalini yoga, nada yoga, etc.) practices to progress the individual along the spiritual path. For instance, integral yoga says that it is essential to practice pranayama yoga to control the breath in order to regulate and soothe the movements of the nervous system, calm the emotions, steady the mind, open the nadi channels and chakras, and retain greater prana force. Although pranayama is a separate yoga practice, it is found within the eight limbs (fourth step) of raja yoga sutras. Both major and minor yogas are complementary to one another, not separate practices. They do not work alone but act as one when blended together in the effort to purify the impediments that hold one back from his or her true identity.

Yoga is a component of many integral spiritual movements to help one progress toward a wholesome spiritual personality.

Chapter 16: Conclusion

In this book I provided you with a comprehensible study of yoga philosopies and ayurveda principles. You can think of these as individual or confluence practices in your spiritual journey to reaching higher states of consciousness. Ultimately, it is up to you to begin or make further progress in your spiritual journey. You are on your way to the final state of liberation or freedom of burden thoughts that weigh your energy and mind down. There are a variety of practices that fit the wide range of personalities, and it is up to the individual to find out what works for him or her. People must determine the particular stage of their spiritual development to overcome the set of circumstances that seem to cause obstacles in their internal and external lives. Learning to endure the adversities in life is very significant to the progress people make along the spiritual journey to realize who they are in relationship to themselves and their circumstances. This is one of the most beautiful features of yoga and ayurveda, and it's what makes them attractive to so many different people. These yogic philosophies and traditions are extremely practical and insightful. People can change their tainted flowers (personality traits) and blossom into the glowing lotus.

Eastern religion and yogic philosophy is conceived as a spiritual journey of the soul through the karmic action and reaction of one's innumerable past and present lifetimes. Similar and definitive circumstances

Dr. John Cosby

arise again and again. These are needed so that we can learn to move on and finalize the crossing over the ocean to the other side, where self-realization awaits. Thus, we can sense that each person's yogic practices are going to be different and require tailor-made techniques and experiences to help guide his or her on his or her spiritual path. All of the yogic practices appear numerous, but essentially, they all aim at accomplishing the same final goal in self-realization.

Over the years I have come to realize that putting aside a set time each day—thirty to forty minutes of meditation and thirty minutes of yoga—has contributed to noteworthy spiritual growth. The addition of other practices, chanting and japa, throughout the day seems to raise sensitivity. Furthermore, the regular attendance at satsanga or maintaining good associations seems to help me realize my actions toward others and help shape me into a better person. I have read countless books on various topics of Eastern philosophy and spoken with a number of qualified teacher to decipher these truths, and they have helped sharpen my intuitivness to knowing myself better and trying to do good with others. I have come to realize that there are many yogic techniques to help the multitude of human personalities in seeking spiritual knowledge. The various styles of yoga can be customized to each individual's emotions, temperament, intellect, and reason. The accumulative effects of the time spent in the practices in order to steady and focus one's mind can enable one to climb

Mind, Ayurveda & Yoga Psychology

the rungs of the ladder to the top, enlightenment. It is well worth the effort.

Each person is fitted to their present spiritual journey as indicated by the samscaras (past impressions), vasanas (subtle desires), and karmas. However, the one common denominator shared by everyone is the power of one's effort to change his or her thought process and to sublimate negative adversities and change them to positive circumstances. But first, aspiration is needed to start up self-effort with genuine sincerity and to lead one to the prosperity of success in every field of life. The failure of event(s) can be attributed to the lack of persistent effort on the part of the individual. Self-effort with endurance is essential to spiritual transformation. The regular practices of yoga and patience allows one to strengthen the will and effort of the mind to overcome any obstacle in life.

Each person is the author to every inscribed circumstance that he or she has encountered. The past effort (or lack of it) is staged under the action of the present conditions. Depending on the past effort of good or bad will it fruitify to the reward and misery of circumstances one has created in their present. Thus, the negativity of the past can be remedied by doing positive self-effort to sublimate the strength of the operating karma. The defects of yesterday can be changed by the effort of today. The endurance of doing good actions will neutralize the past vices and help people live more in accordance to their righteousness, dharma. Sometimes the past iniquity is very strong and continues to prevail over one's current self-effort. One may then ask, "Why is this happening to me?" The lesson here is to endure and accept the unfortunate circumstances by continuing to practice self-effort without hesitation. The persistent effort will eventually defeat the accumulated negative actions of yesterday.

True self-effort is that which promotes joy and sublimate the experience of pain, agony and misery.

Self-Effort (Abhyasa) and Destiny

Most people will attribute their bad circumstances to the concept of destiny. They have given into the idea of destiny to help explain their obstacles in life. They have entertained the idea that "I am reaping the action of my karma that I sowed in the past." They fall to sentiments and rationalization about why they are facing certain painful circumstances. They may even attribute the direction of their life to destiny. They reason that their current circumstances have to happen and by the explanatory action of destiny alone. However, this is only a partial truth, as karma has to be played out, whether good and bad. But apart from destiny, one does have a choice to change past behavior patterns in order to redirect the manifestation of one's present situations. Everyone is given the power to decide what action to take and understanding the consequences that may come with that action. Through willpower, one has the capacity to strengthen self-effort and transcend any circumstance and thus change

Mind, Ayurveda & Yoga Psychology

the concept of destiny. He or she is bound to conquer destiny by the persistent efforts of the yogic disciplines. They can develop spiritual aspiration, inquiry and reflection, discrimination, dispassion, single-minded concentration, and deeper meditation sessions to expand their intuitive intelligence and spontaneity to lead themselves to higher states of consciousness.

In Yoga Vasistha, Sri Jyotirmayanada gives the following illustration:

"An insight into the law of Karma must enable one to discover the innate freedom of the soul to overcome all conditioning circumstances and obstructing conditions. But when one seeks consolation by asserting the law of Karma, he is resigning to a process of inertia."

Final Word to the Book

I would like to end this book with an overview of some very practical things you can do to begin or make progress in your spiritual journey. These are all things that have been discussed in different chapters in the book that I want to emphasize the summation of them here. The regular practice of these instructions can increase spiritual sensitivity and help bring about the integration of one's spiritual personality.

Change your diet. Eating is something we all do every day. Usually more than once! So changing the food you eat can be one of the most profound things you can do to promote physical, mental, and spiritual well-being. There are several different ways one can approach improving one's diet from the perspective of yoga and ayurveda.

First, you can improve your diet by focusing on foods that are sattvic rather than rajasic or tamasic. One should eat more whole foods as opposed to processed or refilled foods. Eat more fresh substances as well as raw and light food instead of heavy and cooked meals. One should eat more fruits, vegetables, nuts, and fresh juices. Juicing has made its way into society in the past few decades. Prepare meals at home instead of eating fast food or foods that come in boxes, cans, or jars. Get to know the properties of foods to maintain your health. For example, eating raw asparagus is a simple way to help cleanse the metals and toxins from the body's circulation and kidney by expelling them through the urinary tract.

Second, one can tailor one's diet according to one's prakruti constitution. The resources in this book can help you to figure out your constitution, or you can consult an ayurvedic physician. Skipping meals or eating less can be a powerful tool in restoring physical health, but understand how to fast the right way. Many if not most diseases are caused by a weak digestive fire, which means that improper foods digested and metabolized turns into ama or toxins. Ayurveda recommends that the stomach be filled halfway with food and one quarter with water. That means one quarter should be left empty. Another ayurvedic principle for eating is said, "Breakfast should be like a king, lunch like a prince, and dinner like a pauper." Ayurveda doesn't traditionally have much to say about midnight snacks, but back then everyone was in bed once it got dark outside! Certainly avoiding nighttime eating can be thought of as a basic principle of ayurveda. Yogis and spiritual practitioners often drastically reduce their food intake or fast for long periods. And it is common practice for spiritually minded aspirants to only eat once a day. But know what you are trying to accomplish. While roughing through the Mumbai region of India, I had the privilege of meeting a Jain monk several times who ate once a day at eleven o'clock in the morning. If he missed eating at that time, he would wait until the next day to eat. It's a little drastic, but you get the point of discipline and self-effort.

And last but not least, the yoga and ayurveda traditions recommend a vegetarian diet as optimal for spiritual, mental, and physical well-being. If you are not already a vegetarian, you might want to consider becoming one or at least reducing your meat consumption, especially in light of the engineering and modififation of meat substances today.

Integrating the Yogic Disciplines

It's through the yogic disciplines of rajas, bhakti, karma, and jnana that one blends the four personality aspects of will, love and devotion, action, and intuitive wisdom to the integration of one's true spirituality.

The essence of every yoga practice is the disciplines

of yama and niyama expounded in raja yoga, which gives an outline to cultivate virtues and avoid vices for the advancement of the spiritual life.

- Cleanliness—purity; clearness of mind, speech, and body.
- Contentment—acceptance of others and of one's circumstances (adversity) as they strengthen one's austerity.
- Study of scripture—listen, contemplate, reflect, and meditate.
- Surrender to God—develop purity of heart.
- Nonviolence—no harm to other living beings.
- Truthfulness—a lack of falsehood.
- Celibacy—not cheating on one's partner.
- Selflessness—no avarice, possessiveness, or theft.

Yoga involves the development of a positive attitude. One does countless activities in life and in turn see these opportunities as chances to be good and do good to advance spiritually. There is no single way but rather innumerable ways in which one can gain virtuous qualities. The cultivation of virtuous qualities replaces characteristic traits so that one can grow into a majestic spiritual personality.

Remember, your thoughts become your actions, and your actions become your habits. And your habits become your character, and your character becomes your effort to change your destiny.

Starting a daily meditation practice is probably the

Mind, Ayurveda & Yoga Psychology

single most powerful thing you can do to transform your life. Studies have shown powerful results from even just a few minutes of meditation a day. All you have to do to start a meditation practice is to sit down in one place and meditate! But there are some things you can do that can be helpful.

It is generally helpful to have a specific time of day that you meditate. Usually, the morning is the best time. In the morning your mind is less active and can more easily settle into deeper states of consciousness. It becomes challenging to shut the mind off and meditate as the day progresses. Moreover, if you plan to develop meditation, it is easier that you do it every day at the same time. Like any learned skill, practice makes perfect.

Setting up a meditation area in your home can be a very useful practice to facilitate meditation. If you have an entire room to use as a separate area for meditation, that is best. A comfortable mat, rug, pillow, and cushion to ease your bodily posture in meditation would be a helpful tool. Pictures, statues, deities, candles, incense, and soft lighting can all be helpful in setting the mood so that you can settle into a deep meditative state. The space should be pleasant to the eyes, relaxing, inspiring, and filled with fresh air to breathe.

The most basic form of meditation is simply sitting in one place and trying to focus one's mind on the mantra sound or on one object. The rhythm of the mantra can be correlated to the length of one's inhale and exhale to slow the respiratory rate of the lungs to

Dr. John Cosby

go deeper into meditation. Attention to breathing can help one counter the random thoughts circulating in the mind. With the rise of attentive thoughts, gently bring your awareness back to your breath and effortlessly repeat the mantra sound to the length and depth of inhalation and exhalation. Other forms of meditation include focusing one's attention on a single point like the flame of a candle or even a picture of one's preferred deity. There are many meditation groups too. Some sit at the shore of the ocean and listen to soft, inspiring sounds of the ways. Others visualize mantra meditation as it transcends consciousness over time. Review the chapter on meditation and see for yourself if you are ready to begin practicing the art of meditation. Remember, posture, breathing, and quiet mindfulness are all important. You can consult Swamiji Joytirmayananda and other highly regarded teachers if you want to learn more about silent meditation or need further guidance.

Start a daily asana practice. This is probably equally as important as meditation, especially given the fact that most people today don't get enough physical activity. Like your meditation practice, it is very useful to have a schedule for your asana practice. You can practice in the morning before meditation, which is best. However, you may want to practice asana yoga during the evening hours since you may have work in the morning.

There are different styles of yoga practice and different asanas that are going to be most beneficial to you, depending on your current physical and mental

Mind, Ayurveda & Yoga Psychology

state and your ayurvedic constitution. You can consult a yoga teacher to help you develop a personal yoga practice, or just experiment and find what works for you. A yoga group class can also be a good way to incorporate a regular yoga practice into your life. Find what works for you!

Start a daily pranayama practice. A pranayama practice naturally complements the discipline of asana and meditation. There are many pranayama exercises one can perform. A simple breathing practice can be done anywhere. You basically sit in one spot and breath in softly and fully through the nose. You pull air into the lower area of the diaphragm (expanding) and exhale softly and fully from the stomach through the nose (contracting). You can do this slowly and deeply several times as your comfort level allows. See chapter 6 for more details. The breathing practice involves attention to the body and mind as well as the softness and gentleness of the rhythmic movement of the lungs. Pranayama is a bridge between the disciplines of asana, meditation, and the mind.

Bhakti yoga (the yoga of devotion) is a profound transformational tool. There are a number of simple things you can do to practice bhakti yoga. The most basic thing you can do is set up an altar in some area of your home. You can do this in your meditation room. Or you can make room in a separate area. Just having an altar somewhere in your home transforms the energy of your home. It brings sattva influence into your home and provides a dose of positive vibration in your life. The more you interact with your altar, the stronger your practice of bhakti yoga will be. Probably the simplest thing you can do is offer incense and flowers to the deity on your altar, which, of course, has an effect on one's consciousness. You can meditate in front of the deity or chant japa on mala beads. You can even put your food in front of your altar to sanctify it before eating. You can practice bhakti yoga to the deity of your choice. You can simply use a picture of a deity. You can use multiple deity statues. Find what images or statues work for you. You can use images from different traditions (i.e., a crucifix or a statue of Buddha). Again, to find what inspires you with devotion, and what imbues your life with grace, beauty, and surrender.

Practice karma yoga. There are various ways one can practice selfless work (karma yoga) as a spiritual discipline. You can give some free time to benefit another or donate money you have earned or commit yourself to a worthy philanthropic cause. You can volunteer time at a charity or religious organization. Ideally, you can find work that inspires you and makes you feel connected to the divine. In our capitalist society, the work we do often alienates us from the divine, but even in alienation and frustration, you can practice being present and doing a good job. Use your work as a time to practice detachment, control of the mind, and being present in the moment. Focus on the little things you can to help others and make a difference in the world, even if your job seems meaningless. And of course, karma yoga doesn't just refer to your job but all the daily activities you do. You can bring spiritual awareness into your romantic relationship or your relationship with your parents or the connection you have with your children, which is a most profound space where you can transform tomorrow's adults.

Jnana yoga is the study of yoga scriptures written by great spiritual teachers like Patanjali Yoga Sutras, Bhagavad-Gita, Yoga Vasistha, and Caraka Samita. The daily practice of reading scriptures reflects a deep spiritual consciousness that can transform one's life. If you are reading this, you are probably already aware that you are a spiritual being and that you should be doing various spiritual practices. Oftentimes we end up doing things we know we shouldn't be doing, falling into old patterns of behavior.

Satsang is another important source of inspiration among spiritually minded people. Take yoga classes at a local yoga studio. Find a local temple, meditation center, or meditation group in your area. The removal of people (thoughtfuless) who are negative influences in your life will only allow steady positive energy into your life. Most important is the shared wisdom from an authentic teacher or guru who has spent most of his or her life reading these great scriptures, which means this person will have an intuitive knowledge of them. Jnana yoga is the accumulation of the living principles of raja yoga, karma yoga, and bhakti yoga and leads to the development of intuitive knowledge, the beginning stage of samadhi.

I wish you all the best in your spiritual journey.

Bibliography

Goswami, Shyam Sundar. *Layayoga: The Definitive Guide to the Chakras and Kundalini.* Rochester, VT: Timer Traditions International, 1999.

Johari, Harish. *Chakras: Energy Centers of Transformation.* Rochester, VT: Destiny Books, 2000.

Kumar, Kamakhya. *Yoga Psychology: A Handbook of Yogic Psychology.* New Dehli, India: D. K. Printworld (P) Ltd., 2013.

Kumar, K. V. Dilip. *Clinical Yoga and Ayurveda.* Dehli: Chaukhamba Sanskrit Pratishthan, 2001.

Mishra, Ramamurti S., MD. *The Textbook of Yoga Psychology.* Baba Bhagavandas Publishing Trust, 1987.

Murthy, Dr. A. R. V. *The Mind in Ayurveda and Other Indian Traditions.* Dehli: Chaukhamba Sanskrit Pratishthan, 2004.

Sharma Priyat Vrat. *Essentials of Ayurveda: Sodasangahrdayam.* Dehli: Motilal Banarsidass Publishers, 1998.

Swami Jyotirmayanada. *Mysteries of the Mind.* Jyotirmayanada Ashram Lalbagh Loni Ghaziabad, U. P. India, 2001.

Swami Jyotirmayanada. *Yoga of Enlightenment*. Yoga Research Foundation, Miami, Fl 33143 USA, 1987.

Swami Jyotirmayanada. *Yoga Vasistha* vol. I–VI. Yoga Research Foundation, Miami, Fl 33143, USA, 1986.

Swami Jyotirmayananda. *Mantra Shiromani*. Yoga Research Foundation, Miami, Fl 33143 USA, 2015.

Swami Satyananda Saraswati. *Asana Pranayama and Mudra Bandha*. Munger, Bihar: Yoga Publications Trust. 1969.

Swami Sivananda. *Raja Yoga*. The Divine Life Society Publications, Himalayas, India 2010.

Swami Sivananda. *Mind: Its Mysteries and Control*. The Divine Life Society Publications, Himalayas, India 2011.

Verma, Vinod. *Ayurveda: A Way of Life*. Samuel Weiser, Inc., Maine, 03902 USA, 1995.

Yogi Ramacharaka. *Science of Breath*. Chicago: Yogi Publicaion Society, 1905.

Woodroffe, Sir John. *Treatise on the Great Liberation*: Ganesh and Company, Madras, India, Reprint 2001.

Autobibliography

Dr. John Cosby received his Bachelor of Arts (B.A.) in Psycholgy from St John's University, New York. He later attended New York Institute of Technology, Long Island, New York, where he received a Master of Science in Training and Learning. His field of specialty was in computer educational software. He graduated with honors. His thesis was a tutorial data base designed for the United States Naval Reserves which was forward by the director of the program to Syracuse University for possible research and implementation of the software. After working for several years he attended medical school at Michigan State University where he received his degree in Doctor of Osteopathic Medicine. He completed his Family Practice Residency at St Barnabas Hospital, Bronx, New York. After completing his residency, he became board certified by the Osteopathic Board of Family Medicine. Thereafter, he opened a family medical clinic in Alachua, Florida, where he began to practice both western medicine and the science of ayuveda.

Prior to medical school, he began to study the science of ayurveda medicine in 1989. His studies of ayurveda lead him to the tutelage of several renown Ayurveda physicians, both in America and India. He was first introduce into Ayurveda by Dr. Vasant Lad at the Ayurvedic Institute, Albuquerque, New Mexico. He continues to take seminars from the Dr. Lad to further his studies in ayurveda. Dr. Cosby realized the implementation of the two medicine, western and eastern, offered a powerful and synergistic form of medicine to his patients. He combined ayurveda herbal formulas and detoxification programs, and the usage of limited pharmaceutical medicine at his clinic when needed with positive results.

His passion for the holistic approach of ayurveda lead him to give seminars of the ancient knowknowledge to practitioners and individual for the purpose of self-healing thyself.

Throughout his spiritual journey and ayuveda, he has realized the root of every disease can be attributed to the manifestation of some imbalance in the mind. As result, his medical practice has developed into consultation in yoga psychology, implementation of ayurveda herbs for the mind, classes and seminars, counseling in proper nutrition and lifestyle of body type, and a second coming book on Vedanta and the Unconscious Mind.

Dr. John Cosby can be reached through the email of ayurvedic4free@yahoo.com

Lightning Source UK Ltd.
Milton Keynes UK
UKHW041929101122
411987UK00001B/201